The Practice Development Unit:
An experiment in multidisciplinary innovation

The Practice Development Unit: An experiment in multidisciplinary innovation

Edited by
Steve Page RGN, BA (Hons), MSc
David Allsopp RGN, BSc (Hons), MA
Sally Casley RGN, RM, DMS, FETC

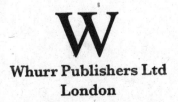

Whurr Publishers Ltd
London

© 1998 Whurr Publishers Ltd
First published 1998 by
Whurr Publishers Ltd
19b Compton Terrace, London N1 2UN, England

Reprinted 2000 and 2003

British Library Cataloguing in Publication Data
A catalogue record for this book is available from the
British Library.

ISBN 1 86156 052 4

Contents

v

Part II: The PDU in practice

Contributors

Editors and major contributors

David Allsopp RGN, BSc (Hons), MA Lecturer in Nursing, School of Nursing, Midwifery and Health Visiting, Manchester University. Formerly Research Practitioner, Practice Development Unit, Seacroft Hospital, Leeds.

Sally Casley RGN, RM, DMS, FETC Deputy Head, Effective Practice Unit, St. James's and Seacroft University Hospitals NHS Trust, Leeds. Formerly Practice Development Unit Leader, Seacroft Hospital, Leeds, 1996–1997.

Debbie Lee RGN, DipN, CIM, MBA Nursing Officer, Department of Health. Formerly Patient Services Manager/Practice Development Unit Director, Seacroft Hospital, Leeds.

Mike Lowry RGN, B.Ed.(Hons), RNT, M.Ed, PGCRM Senior Lecturer in Nursing, Leeds Metropolitan University.

Hugo Mascie-Taylor FRCP (Lond), FRCPI, MHSM, A.DipC. Director of Commissioning, Leeds Health Authority. Formerly Consultant Physician – Medicine for the Elderly /Practice Development Unit Director, Seacroft Hospital, Leeds.

Steve Page RGN, BA (Hons), MSc Directorate Head of Nursing – Surgery, Royal Victoria Infirmary and Associated Hospitals NHS Trust, Newcastle upon Tyne. Formerly Practice Development Unit Leader, Seacroft Hospital, Leeds, 1994–1996.

Angela Turner RGN, RSCN, FETC, PG Dip – Quality Assurance and Social Care Director of Nursing Services – Surgery, Kingsmill Centre for Health Services, Notts. Formerly Programme Director, Institute of Nursing at Leeds University.

Additional contributors

Chapters 1 and 2

Carol Williams Assistant Director of Nursing, Cornwall Healthcare Trust. Original Practice Development Unit Leader.

Chapter 6

Jane Farley Ward Manager, Practice Development Unit, Seacroft Hospital.
Lynn George Senior Dietitian, Seacroft Hospital.

Chapter 7

Janis Brown Staff Nurse, Practice Development Unit, Seacroft Hospital.
Cathy Lowe Senior Pharmacist, Pharmacy Academic Practice Unit, Leeds University. Formerly Senior Pharmacist, Seacroft Hospital.

Chapter 8

Gwen Al-Khaili Clinical Sister, Chapel Allerton Hospital. Formerly Staff Nurse, Practice Development Unit, Seacroft Hospital.
Karen Atkinson Ward Sister, St James's Hospital. Formerly Staff Nurse, Practice Development Unit, Seacroft Hospital.
Tracy Cloke Ward Manager, Practice Development Unit, Seacroft Hospital.
Mary Dawson Formerly Senior Occupational Therapist, Seacroft Hospital (now retired).
Aiden Devlin Clinical Support Worker, Practice Development Unit, Seacroft Hospital.
Jane Farley Ward Manager, Practice Development Unit, Seacroft Hospital.
Pat Fletcher Senior Physiotherapist, Seacroft Hospital.
June Lancaster Divisional Manager/Senior Nurse, Trauma related Services, St James's Hospital. Formerly Hospital Services Manager/Practice Development Unit Director, Seacroft Hospital.
Mandy Phelan-Oldfield Ward Manager, Practice Development Unit, Seacroft Hospital.

Charlie Teale Consultant Physician – Medicine for the Elderly, Seacroft Hospital.

Chapter 9

Liz Hayward Ward Manager, Seacroft Hospital.

Chris Patterson Senior Registrar, St James's Hospital. Formerly Senior Registrar, Seacroft Hospital.

Irene Waddington Formerly Staff Nurse, Practice Development Unit, Seacroft Hospital (now retired).

Chapter 10

Nicky David Ward Sister, St James's Hospital. Formerly Ward Sister, Seacroft Hospital.

Mandy Phelan-Oldfield Ward Manager, Practice Development Unit, Seacroft Hospital.

Preface

The Practice Development Unit (PDU) was established to provide a focus within its hospital for multidisciplinary practice development and research, and to support dissemination of innovation.

The Seacroft unit was the originator of the model, which was developed as a result of dissatisfaction with the capacity of the Nursing Development Unit approach to address the multidisciplinary nature of health care. Although originally differences between the two approaches were only vaguely defined, after six years of continued development, significant differences are now apparent in their philosophy, focus and organisation of work, and potential benefits.

Key among these differences is the extent to which the PDU operates beyond the confines of a unidisciplinary focus, and addresses the pressing need to break down barriers and tackle issues at the interfaces of practice – between disciplines, between clinical staff and managers, between hospital and community, between academics and practitioners. This facility uniquely equips the PDU to deal with many of the current clinical and managerial priorities in the health service, as well as remaining an effective vehicle for development within the professional disciplines.

Within its own organisation, the PDU has brought about significant culture change and numerous developments which have been freely shared. This has resulted in an impact on quality of patient care which is well recognised both inside and outside the hospital; and the unit has been acknowledged as a key resource for the organisation as a whole.

The unit and its activity have been publicised via journal and conference papers, and substantial reference has been made to its work by external authors. However, the PDU has now reached a stage where it seems appropriate to examine its work in more detail, to present a more comprehensive view of its operation, and to share the wealth of the team's experience with others. To this end it seemed timely to consider the production of this book.

Our intention is to offer an understanding of the theoretical basis of the PDU model and its application to practice, as well as insight into the benefits and complexities of the approach. We are not seeking to promote the PDU as a universal panacea, nor suggesting that the approach described should be applied in every detail. Rather, the focus of the book on real practical issues is intended to offer genuine insight into the implementation and continued support of such a unit, as well as the often severe difficulties of maintaining its work in the face of external pressures and conflicting organisational cultures. It is intended to offer clear pointers as to how the general principles might be adapted to suit differing circumstances, as a powerful means of taking practice forward.

The PDU has received a steady stream of enquiries and visits, both from teams interested in developing their own PDU and from individuals involved in broader developmental work. The content of the book reflects real concerns and questions raised by such visitors as well as the reflections of practitioners within the PDU itself. We hope, therefore, that it will be a useful resource for a wide range of professionals from any discipline, including clinical staff, practice developers, researchers, educationalists, audit and quality improvement practitioners, and leaders/managers seeking to get the best from their teams.

Introduction

The development and evaluation of professional health care practice has historically been undertaken largely along unidisciplinary lines, with little attention being paid to the interfaces between disciplines. The implementation of general management principles over recent years, however, has brought with it a sharper focus on the quality and efficiency of the whole service, and this has left us in little doubt that many of the issues adversely affecting quality and efficiency are related precisely to these interfaces, and to the barriers between different disciplines and departments.

The current agenda for health service development is increasingly dominated by a small number of issues, including the need for increased patient-centred care and user involvement, emphasis on clinical audit and clinical effectiveness, and concerns about efficiency and value for money. In order to respond effectively to these new challenges, a new approach is needed which goes beyond a narrow unidisciplinary focus and truly reflects the multidisciplinary, multiagency nature of health care provision.

Many of the changes made since the introduction of general management have been designed to break down traditional professional boundaries, and to facilitate the examination of practice across disciplines and departments. However, it could be argued that these often tend towards genericism, with the resultant danger that input from the various clinical professions can be undervalued. Frequently the plans of managers and clinical professionals are not effectively integrated, so that the planning of new developments is inefficient and uncoordinated. Worse still, management has been perceived by some (Ford and Walsh 1994) as another emerging profession, which in itself can dominate the practice of others and warp the priorities of the health care team.

There is a need, therefore, to develop an approach to practice which not only reflects the multidisciplinary nature of our service, but at the same time facilitates the link between clinicians and managers and ensures that the unique contribution of each professional discipline is not lost in the drive for greater efficiency. Many initiatives can be identified which address some of these needs, such as quality improvement programmes, development of clinical audit, involvement of clinical staff in business planning, and Nursing Development Unit (NDU) schemes. At Seacroft Hospital, however, a unique approach was developed which we feel affects all of these areas.

The Practice Development Unit (PDU) was established around the base of four wards in a medical/elderly unit, with the purpose of supporting multidisciplinary practice development and research, and of disseminating ideas and innovations. The principles underpinning the unit included an emphasis on a multidisciplinary approach, empowerment of patients, staff development and establishment of an open management culture supporting the involvement of all staff and ensuring that those closest to patients were leading or actively involved in new developments. While having some similarities to the NDU framework, the new approach also drew on various other sources – such as management theory related to quality improvement, change and teamwork. Added together, however, we believe that this combination was significantly greater than the sum of its parts, and represented a new approach uniquely suited to meeting the newly emerging priorities of the health service.

Since its establishment, the unit has grown and produced work of increasing sophistication and benefit to its patients. It has been successful in developing and disseminating new practice, with many new developments impacting directly on the quality or cost-effectiveness of patient care.

The unit has not remained unaltered, however, but has evolved in response to changing circumstances and priorities around it. Surrounded by massive organisational change, it has proved itself to be both resilient and extremely adaptable – continuing to produce and see through innovations in spite of the uncertainty surrounding it.

The structure and support of the unit have developed, together with a far clearer view of its philosophy and distinguishing features.

Most importantly, the unit has developed extremely effective approaches to the dissemination of new work, and to integration of the work of the clinical and managerial teams, to ensure that the work of the unit is not seen as a mere luxury or optional extra, but is seen as integral to the organisation as a whole.

This book begins with a discussion of the unit's original inception, its background and the emergence of the new model. The practical steps taken to realise this are examined in some detail, as well as the obstacles encountered and how they were overcome. While the circumstances surrounding the emergence of any unit are unique, it is hoped that the principles underlying the PDU approach and many of the practical measures adopted will be readily transferable to other settings.

The new model and its key principles are described in detail, with subsequent chapters discussing the continued evolution of the model and its support systems. One chapter is exclusively devoted to an exploration of the differences between PDUs and NDUs. We feel that this emphasis is justified for two main reasons. Firstly, because although there are many easily identifiable similarities between the two approaches, there is a lack of conceptual clarity generally as to their differences, together with a tendency to consider the two types of unit to be synonymous in practice. The second reason is a desire to demonstrate the distinct benefits of the PDU approach, lying in its operation beyond the unidisciplinary level.

The second half of the book takes up the key principles expounded in the earlier chapters, devoting a separate chapter to each to examine its significance in more detail and to demonstrate, by reference to a variety of project work, how each has been fulfilled. We have sought to demonstrate the relevance of PDU activity to the needs of patients and carers, and to those of the hospital as a whole. Input from current and former members of the team describing their own experiences and how working in the PDU has affected their approach to work and career development complements this section, to illustrate the central importance to the PDU's success of developing and empowering its staff.

The final chapter addresses the issue of evaluation. We have gathered a considerable quantity of information to evaluate both the impact of specific project work and the quality and cost-effectiveness of the unit as a whole. Increasingly, the unit is seeking direct input from patients and other users, as well as from the individual members of the team, to enrich this evaluative process with more qualitative data. Examples of this work are discussed, and also the complexities of undertaking it. There is a recognition of the need to undertake a more rigorous and objective evaluation of the PDU, and this section therefore also considers the complex issues involved in implementing a multisite research study of the PDU approach, involving units at different stages of development. Finally, this section will also seek to review the impact of the unit in broader terms on those around it, both within its own organisation and beyond.

In structuring the book in this way, we hope to be able to demonstrate the theoretical underpinning of the unit, and also to show clearly how this theoretical model is realised, providing a resource for any others wishing to pursue the PDU approach, as well as for those wishing to investigate approaches to development of multidisciplinary practice in more general terms. In addition, the specific developmental work used to illustrate the PDU principles relates to issues of common concern, and hopefully will provide considerable food for thought in itself.

The PDU has had a difficult history, needing to adapt constantly to changes in external circumstances in order to survive. It has weathered at least four major upheavals in its hospital management over the last six years and as this book was being written, the effects of the latest of these – a merger with a large teaching hospital trust – were beginning to have a serious impact on the function of the unit. This new organisational environment is characterised by traditional professional and departmental demarcations and styles of working which are often in direct conflict with the philosophy and methods of the PDU itself, and at this stage it is unlikely that the unit will continue to survive in its current form. The crucial importance of long-term, active support from senior managers of the wider organisation for the unit's culture and its work will therefore be examined in some detail. Nevertheless, even in this context, the influence of the PDU and its team on trust-wide developments in clinical effectiveness, quality improvement and clinical audit is recognised and this in itself may lead to a new phase for the unit, with different modes of working adapted to suit its new situation.

We therefore see this book as merely the starting point for examination of the PDU approach. As the unit continues to evolve, and as other units currently embarking progress further, more will be understood about what makes for a successful PDU, and we expect that the groundwork laid out in this book will be built on.

We hope also that this book will contribute to debates about issues such as multidisciplinary practice development, patient-centred care, integration of the clinical and managerial agenda and clinical effectiveness. In particular, we feel that it has something to say on the subject of implementing change in a multidisciplinary clinical environment. Even in the midst of the growing emphasis on evidence-based practice, the complexities of the clinical setting and necessary sophistication of the change process needed to overcome these, tend to be overlooked in favour of the development of new research and publication in different forms of the results.

Finally, this book is written in the spirit of the PDU itself – one of openness in expressing new ideas, a genuine desire to share these with others and to explore how they can be developed further. We hope that you will enjoy reading our ideas and experiences, but that these will also stimulate discussion and new developments in your own areas which will enrich your practice and benefit both patients and staff. Equally, we hope that the ensuing debates will help us to enhance our own practice, so that we too can continue to grow.

Part I
Development and
Support of the
Practice
Development Unit

Chapter 1
Origins of the Practice Development Unit: an approach to radical change in a multidisciplinary setting

David Allsopp, Debbie Lee and
Hugo Mascie-Taylor

Historical roots of the Practice Development Unit

The Seacroft Practice Development Unit (PDU) has been in existence for five years. It has been an interesting and at times challenging period, during which there have been several major changes brought about by the NHS reforms:

- The PDU has had to adjust to changes in bed usage resulting in the closure of one of its four wards.
- It has expanded to include the rest of the Department of Medicine (a change which is still being worked through).
- It has seen the department itself merged into a larger Division of Medicine which spans two sites three miles apart.
- It has seen changes in its leadership.

Seacroft Hospital has during the same period undergone several reorganisations as it has worked with four different hospitals in and around Leeds at various times. The hospital has become part of a relatively enormous NHS trust with a very different culture. Change, as they say, is here to stay.

Even to think about setting up a practice development unit during such a time would strike many as asking too much of people. Yet it is our belief that the PDU has helped us to adapt and survive. It has helped to raise the profile of Seacroft Hospital when to some there were serious questions about its future, and has helped to motivate staff who understandably felt pressured by all the changes. Above all it has shown those working in it that they can be effective in changing practice for the better. It has demonstrated that staff not previously used to influencing change can do so, and make a good job of it.

The emphasis on multidisciplinary working is a key feature of the PDU and is what sets it apart from other development units. There are particular historical reasons for this, which will be explained in this chapter. The lessons for others are less about taking this model of practice development and using it in their own setting, and more about seeing what is possible if health care staff pull together instead of in different directions.

The key questions are how to work most effectively with colleagues and to ask 'who is relevant to this problem?' Everyone needs to work together in achieving common aims in the interests of patients and other users of health services. There are very few issues which are the concern of one profession only. Delivering effective health care is not just about giving the right treatment, it is about the whole team working together to ensure a quality service. We need to understand each other's roles and how they are complementary and overlap. We need to think creatively and be imaginative in finding new solutions to old problems. Above all we need to make sure that any changes we make are truly in the interests of those whom we serve, our patients.

The aims of this chapter are to describe the origins of the Seacroft Practice Development Unit and to analyse the factors which supported its inception. In particular it will show how the special circumstances of the closure of one hospital and the subsequent transfer of its services for the elderly to another site were relevant to the creation of the PDU. These events were significant in providing a wonderful opportunity to apply knowledge of management and organisational theory in a way that was constructive and supportive.

St George's Hospital: roots of the PDU

The idea for a practice development unit first arose in 1991 when plans were being made to transfer a service for the elderly from St George's Hospital on the edge of Leeds to Seacroft Hospital, seven miles away. St George's would then be closed down. Most of the patients at St George's needed extended or respite care or long term rehabilitation. There were relatively few patients with acute medical problems. This was partly because St George's lacked the necessary support services and discharging patients to other settings was at the time given a low priority. For many patients, and perhaps for some staff too, St George's was like home. It certainly had a friendly, community atmosphere which is sometimes lost in more acute settings. Often more than one family member would work somewhere within the hospital. This gave the hospital a family feel, and, as in many families, members would fall out occasionally but in times of hardship or trouble they would pull together. Staff were very flexible. It was not unusual for someone to come into work at very short notice if there was sudden sickness, or if a ward became very busy someone would pop in to help for a few hours. The porters, for example, would not only undertake the duties expected of them but also ran the switchboard. They would mop the floor if they came across any spillages. 'Multiskilling' was part of the subconscious. It was important to try and preserve as much as possible of these attitudes. This became harder than anticipated, as teams were inevitably broken up, or merged into larger teams of Seacroft staff.

Many of the staff lived in the local area, often within walking distance, although patients came from all over Leeds. Morale was reasonably high although among some of the staff there was a feeling that they were very much 'second best' to those in the teaching hospitals. The hospital had been administered by both major Leeds hospitals over the years and by 1990 was the responsibility of the local health authority as part of a directly managed unit which included Seacroft Hospital, with which it was to merge.

Seacroft Hospital

Seacroft Hospital had for many years been linked with St James's University Hospital but had parted ways when the larger partner became a first wave Trust in 1992. As well as elective surgical work, the general medical and infectious diseases wards admitted acute patients directly from the local community. A cystic fibrosis unit was also very active. Within the Department of Medicine there were three consultant general physicians with individual speciality interests and a cardiologist. Generally, morale amongst Seacroft staff was high and the hospital enjoyed a good reputation for its services. Although larger than St George's, Seacroft also had something of a small community feel to it.

Merger of Seacroft and St George's Hospitals

The rationale for the merger was partly saving money – St George's was a large, open site, expensive to maintain – and partly political – it was government policy to close down long-term hospital care and encourage the development of private nursing home care as an alternative.

The plan was to move the five remaining wards at St George's into a new medical block together with the existing acute medical wards already in old accommodation at Seacroft. The new Department of Medicine would have a non-age-related admissions policy, and the service would be fully integrated, with therapy support from physiotherapists, occupational therapists and others actually based in the department as close to patients as possible. In this sense there was a real attempt to develop a 'patient focused service', organised around the needs of patients, and less around the needs of the service providers.

The plan was greeted by staff at St George's with varying degrees of enthusiasm as one might expect. For some it raised real fears about changes in roles, about the need for a different set of skills. Many staff had worked at St George's for many years and felt extremely threatened by the change, thinking they lacked the necessary skills and that their patients would be neglected in wards that dealt with acutely ill people of all ages.

There was also a concern that the shift in focus away from specifically elderly care would damage years of hard work in promoting the specialist needs of older people in hospital. A fear that older people with chronic illness and requiring rehabilitation would be marginalised as younger patients competed for beds was later proved to be unfounded, as more than 70% of admissions were over 65 years of age. Many younger patients benefited from having ward based rehabilitation and older patients benefited from acute specialist care.

For some the changes were too much. Some took the opportunity for early retirement and some left soon after the move, feeling that life at Seacroft was just not the same. Other staff saw the merger as an opportunity for professional development which had previously eluded them and which would provide their patients with a better quality service.

Most of the consultants involved with St George's transferred not to Seacroft, but to the St James's University Hospital, shortly to become a first wave NHS Trust. The irony was that Seacroft would later merge with St James's, raising new questions about the provision of medical and elderly services and challenging the practice development approach so carefully nurtured in its infancy at St George's.

As the time approached for the move to Seacroft, fears continued to develop and morale fell. The managerial challenge was to raise morale, increase levels of confidence and to develop amongst staff a range of technical skills which would be necessary in the care of acutely ill patients.

What were the aims of setting up the PDU?

By 1990 St George's Hospital had been without an on-site manager for over a year. In some ways this was a problem in dealing with operational issues and did not help in making staff feel a valued part of the larger organisation. In other ways it meant that staff had to become fairly self-sufficient and to take responsibility much more than those working in other settings might have been used to. It is to their credit that staff remained fully committed to quality patient care despite the lack of direct support and direction. It also helps to explain how ways of working which were much more patient centred were able to develop: there was no real opposition to any proposals for change from higher authorities. Such a sense of autonomy, once acquired, is difficult to lose and was carried forward to Seacroft. When in later years the PDU was to become part of a much larger hospital trust with a rather different organisational culture, there were some difficulties as well as advantages. These are discussed in chapter 12.

Opportunities for change

The merger of the St George's elderly and Seacroft medical wards into one integrated department of medicine presented opportunities for change, with all the consultant staff acting as general physicians with particular interests, and all the wards taking unselected general medical patients. The advantages of this approach for patients was that they would reap the benefits of access to expertise from both elderly and acute medical traditions. This was not just about medical skills, but nursing and therapy skills too. The relatively small size (around 174 beds, including six coronary care beds) of the merged department made an integrated department more manageable. There were also advantages in sharing junior medical staffing. The integrated service would be distinctly different from other medical and elderly services in the city, which would appeal to purchasing authorities.

Creating a new merged department was a major piece of organisational development which involved considerable discussion and debate between the staff from both sites. It was part of the management style to be as open as possible and to involve staff at all levels in these discussions. It was seen as important that all had the opportunity to express their fears about the merger and discuss solutions to problems freely. One approach was to hold 'time out' sessions, with as many present as possible from all occupations and grades, whilst keeping the service running. These were invaluable in breaking down barriers, enabling people to get to know each other and understand concerns. They were to continue to be useful (although there is obviously a limit to how often you can hold them) in developing ideas for the PDU.

The relevance of nursing development units (NDUs)

One of the ideas discussed before the merger was setting up a nursing development unit (NDU). It was thought this might provide the sort of stimulus required to motivate staff to feel positive about the move. The opportunity to bid for large grants of up to £100 000 from the King's Fund to support NDUs was approaching, and it was tempting to apply.

Although many of the values and aspirations of NDUs were consistent with our own, one of the earliest decisions made was to establish a practice development unit (PDU) rather than a nursing development unit. The idea of an NDU was rejected because of the strong multidisciplinary ethos which existed at St George's and which is a common feature of elderly care services. The emphasis upon the development of one profession was inappropriate in a multidisciplinary team. A more detailed discussion of the main differences between NDUs and the Seacroft PDU follows in Chapter 5. For now, it is important simply to acknowledge the influence of NDUs on the early thinking about the Seacroft PDU.

The emergence of nursing development units in the 1980s was a sign that it was possible to start challenging the existing NHS culture, by daring to take the lead in trying new approaches to health care. It is interesting to note that the first NDUs tended to be associated with elderly care settings, where the dominance of medicine was perhaps less strong (though nonetheless real). This provided opportunities for those wishing for a more assertive role (such as nurses) to take the initiative. The NDU movement has done much to raise the confidence of nurses in promoting the value of their contribution to health care.

Visiting NDUs was useful in helping to clarifying ideas and giving something with which to compare approaches. The more the team thought about it the more obvious it became that the multidisciplinary model of a practice development unit felt right. It seems incredible now how much effort was put into thinking what to call the unit, but it has to be remembered that there was no other PDU model and that there were only NDUs to relate to. It was important to be clear about how a PDU differed from an NDU beyond saying that it was just multidisciplinary. NDUs had a commitment to 'close relationships with other health staff', but it was felt that this was not enough.

Developing a patient focus

Another influence on early thinking in developing the PDU philosophy was the work being done on 'patient focused care' in the USA. This is an approach which attempts to place the patient truly in the centre of events, instead of organising services so that functions are centralised away from the patient. It is a common feature of modern hospitals that patients are cared for in wards, but are hauled off to other departments such as X-ray or physiotherapy for investigations or treatment. A patient focused approach asks if this is really necessary. Obviously it does not make sense to have an operating theatre on every ward, but bringing other services such as physiotherapy and occupational therapy to the ward can make a difference. We were fortunate at Seacroft to be able to provide treatment rooms actually on the wards. This had the benefit of making it easy to transfer patients to treatment rooms. It also meant that therapy staff were much more visible on the ward and their presence meant they could be seen for what they were: true members of the multidisciplinary team. However, being patient focused is not just a matter of bringing services geographically closed to patients. It is also about doing things differently and having a different attitude to service delivery. Whenever a change to a service is considered, the driving question should be 'what is in the best interests of patients?' Sometimes this is forgotten, and services are organised to suit the needs of the providers rather than the users of a service.

For example, physiotherapists required a written referral from a doctor before they could see a patient and assess the need for treatment. This process would involve first of all the decision to refer; this would be made sometimes by the consultant or other doctor on a ward round, and at other times by a nurse, who would ask a junior doctor to sign a referral form which would be sent through internal mail to the physio department. It could take up to three working days from sending the referral form to the patient being assessed for treatment. Instead, agreement was reached enabling nurses to refer for physiotherapy assessment on the basis of trigger factor criteria. Doctors could still refer in the old way if necessary, but the nurse now had the advantage of being able to refer directly when she saw the physio on the ward. Referral to contact time was cut dramatically, saving time and getting treatment to patients much more quickly. The old approach of needing a referral form because the system required it was thrown out, to be replaced with a service much more responsive to the needs of patients.

Moving to Seacroft gave a real opportunity to look at the ways of delivering patient care. The basic principle was to group things together based on the requirements of the patients. For this it was necessary to review the training of staff, the structure of care teams, the use of practice guidelines, operational policies, protocols and multidisciplinary standards. Placing the patient truly at the centre of events was seen as a way of decreasing delays, disruption and inconvenience, while increasing the clarity about who was caring for them and improving the organisation of the patient's day.

How were the changes achieved?

Creation of the practice development unit involved a profound cultural change. There were several features of organisational culture that it was necessary to change if the PDU was to be successful. A key aspect of the change in culture seen at St George's was a shift from being part of an organisation which put up barriers to every suggested change, to one where there was a real commitment to continuous quality improvement. The traditional structures of NHS hospitals are somewhat hierarchical and bureaucratic – what Handy (1985) describes as **role cultures**. The features of a role culture are that it has departments or functions that are clearly defined, within which people work in set roles. Roles are defined by job descriptions and there are set procedures for communication and for the settlement of disputes. People are not expected to perform beyond the requirements of their role, and in fact this may be actively discouraged. Power in such organisations is associated with roles, what Handy calls 'position power', and the way to influence change is through rules and procedures. Role cultures are controlled and coordinated from the top by senior managers. Everything works well as long as departments do their defined jobs and people perform according to their roles. It is a rational system which is often successful operating in stable environments.

Where role cultures have more difficulty is in responding to constantly changing circumstances. As Handy says, they 'are slow to perceive the need for change and slow to change even if the need is seen' (p. 191).

Often, organisations – especially large hospital trusts – are much more complex than this description suggests. Included also are elements of what Handy refers to as a **person culture**, in which individuals are seen as a central focus. The organisation exists to serve the needs of that individual around whom everything seems to revolve. Most health service workers will be familiar with examples of consultants who operate in this way. Having a person culture within a role culture can make management a demanding task, and also makes it difficult for others within an organisation who wish to influence change.

The sort of culture which seemed best suited to the rapidly changing demands created by the closure of St George's Hospital and the merger with Seacroft was the **task culture**. This is one which is much more flexible and adaptable than a role culture, which places a heavy emphasis upon 'getting the job done'. Project teams or groups are set up to tackle particular tasks and there is much more of an egalitarian feel to things. Teamwork is important and it does not matter who is involved in a project, as long as they have the right skills and are at the most appropriate level. Responsibility is passed 'downwards' and the importance of expert power is recognised. Task cultures are more often associated with small organisations, which probably explains some of the difficulties faced by the PDU in later years, as it merged with a large hospital trust. Task cultures are difficult to control and when resources are constrained, as they always are in the health service, there is a tendency to revert to a role culture.

The management style at both St George's and Seacroft was one which was sympathetic to the task culture model. This did not mean that existing hierarchies were completely overturned. To achieve this would be an enormous task which would involve a complete review of the roles of professionals and the ways they related to each other. This was not the aim. Rather, it was a more modest one of encouraging the view that staff could be more effective in helping patients if they worked closely together in solving problems. The boundary between professions was particularly important, for it is here that issues of team work and communication arise. In a department of medicine dealing with the needs of a largely elderly client group, it is hard to think of an issue which is not of concern to a range of professional or service providers.

Leadership approach

The patient services manager, clinical nurse specialist and clinical director saw it as a joint responsibility to assist the process of change. Values of openness, a desire to involve others in the change process, to devolve responsibility 'downwards' (nearer to the patient), a commitment to improving patient care and to multidisciplinary forms of working were values shared by all three. Aims were clear and the support of staff was sought in achieving them. The key task was developing a service that could compete in the future, which had built-in strategic flexibility. It was perceived that the survival of the service was dependent on a major transformation of the way in which things were done.

The first thing was to create a vision of how the service could look. Staff obviously needed to share that vision and be committed to it and it was vital that any changes became established as part of the organisation culture. The removal of fear and low self-esteem was an urgent task. The best way of tackling this was by being as open and honest as possible with everyone and by persuading staff to realise the value of their work. PDU leaders needed to be clear about what was negotiable and what was not. Recognised change strategies of involving people at an early stage and developing ownership of the problem were essential to this process. By seeking to promote increased responsibility through discussions of roles, the functions of primary nursing teams and how they related to other professions and the involvement of key stakeholders, we hoped to overcome some of the difficulties.

Building the vision

Historically much work had been carried out at St George's Hospital to provide a multidisciplinary approach to care, with the emphasis being placed on the patient as the focus of all activity. The multidisciplinary team of nurses, doctors, physiotherapists and occupational therapists, with clerical support from the ward clerks, was supported by social workers, dietitians, pharmacists, speech therapists and a chiropodist.

Effective multidisciplinary teams are not unique, but to adapt successfully to rapid change everyone was going to have to pull together in their response to new challenges and opportunities.

Much of the discussion in the weekly multidisciplinary meetings focused around sharing information and news of the move and letting off steam about any operational issues. There was also much debate about how the service should develop and many ideas were considered, including the restructuring of care teams, the decentralisation of services bringing them as close as possible to the patient's bedside and multiskilling of staff for the delivery of routine procedures rather than referral to a specialist.

Staff needed to feel a sense of ownership of the changes. This would only happen if they had opportunities to participate and feel valued. As well as the meetings there were occasional workshops, held when possible off the hospital site and in an environment where staff could relax and have the space to think and debate in small groups.

For many of the staff the opportunity to discuss their work in this way was a very new experience and one which could be at times quite challenging. Terms like 'SWOT' and 'PEST' became more familiar. For some it was quite difficult to get used to the idea of openly talking about the strengths and weaknesses of the service in front of senior staff. Similarly, being asked to think about and comment on organisational politics was totally new. There is always a danger here of alienating people through the use of language that is unfamiliar and strange. It is vital that such jargon is avoided as much as possible. Instead, it is the principles that matter: those of listening, respecting each other's views, being able to accept reasonable criticism and avoidance of blame.

In such times of change effective communication is vital. Apart from meeting on a very regular basis to share views and news, informal communication by walking the patch was also helpful.

Figure 1.1 illustrates the route taken in establishing the PDU. Early work on multidisciplinary standard setting was invaluable in bringing professions together and agreeing on a package of care that best met patient need. There were considerable benefits in developing understanding of each other's roles and how they fitted together. This did much to cement the team together. It was important that there was clarity of role within teams, with staff valuing each other. Such discussions were especially useful in building confidence, since the more staff talked with each other about what they contributed, the more each valued what they did. Such open discussion is perhaps a rare luxury in which health care teams indulge too little. The day-to-day pressures of work make it difficult to find the time to discuss anything other than immediate clinical issues. Teams can then lose sight of their objectives and become less effective in delivering care. The period of preparation for the merger provided a wonderful stimulus to the process of reviewing team values and objectives, structures and processes and was fundamental to the development of the PDU philosophy.

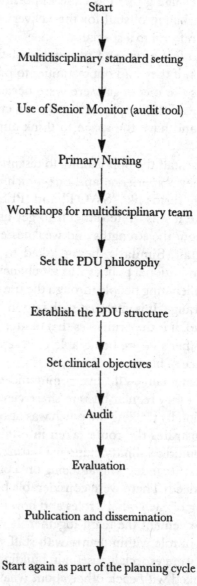

Start

↓

Multidisciplinary standard setting

↓

Use of Senior Monitor (audit tool)

↓

Primary Nursing

↓

Workshops for multidisciplinary team

↓

Set the PDU philosophy

↓

Establish the PDU structure

↓

Set clinical objectives

↓

Audit

↓

Evaluation

↓

Publication and dissemination

↓

Start again as part of the planning cycle

Figure 1.1. Route to becoming a Practice Development Unit

The most important factors

There were several factors which it was important to work on if the PDU was to break down some of the barriers to effective team working which the old style NHS seemed to present.

Structure

The first of these was structure. The move to primary nursing encouraged nurses to take more responsibility for care decisions than they had perhaps been used to. Primary nurses were asked to take on the task of deciding on the need for referral to therapists, according to clear criteria set out by the therapists. This had the effect of speeding the referral process so that patients were assessed and treated by, say, a physiotherapist more quickly. Doctors were relieved of the requirement to complete a referral form, and nurses were empowered to make decisions for themselves. This did not rule out doctors being involved, as they were still made aware that referrals had taken place. Primary nurses were also expected to attend ward rounds for their patients instead of the sister (the traditional approach). This encouraged more involvement and discussion with doctors and others on the rounds and in team meetings. It also raised the profile of primary nurses in the eyes of consultants and did much to encourage the view that knowledge and expertise were perhaps more important than status or role.

In addition, the PDU moved away from seeing problem solving as something only for senior staff, to recognising that the problem is often best understood by those dealing with it every day. Involving junior staff in project teams was one way of acknowledging the contribution that staff could make quite successfully to practice development.

Responsibility

Involving staff not normally used to project work gives them a sense of responsibility which empowers and develops them.

Risk

Allowing staff more responsibility to solve their own problems involves a certain amount of risk taking, as one can never be sure what the outcome will be. What remains important is that potential risks are considered and that careful planning takes place to minimise risk. One risk is that projects are not completed and that problems remain unresolved. This highlights the need to agree clear project objectives for which group leaders can be held accountable.

Support

The experience of staff at St George's was that senior management were perceived as rather distant, not helped by their total absence from the site for a period. Distance is not just geographical, but is also achieved by management style. It was necessary that support for staff was clear and visible, and was enacted not just nominal. This was accomplished by having a clear support structure, with a PDU leader to coordinate activities, a quality assurance nurse to help with audit and evaluation, a research advisory group to support research and various opportunities for staff to express views at open management meetings. A process of individual performance review was also encouraged which sought to link objectives with ward and team objectives. The PDU Steering Group was also valuable in giving senior management support to the initiative.

Standards

The approach to standard setting was at first often uniprofessional, with little consideration of the need to take a wider view. This was perhaps necessary as professionals learnt the techniques of setting standards and gained experience of audit. It became increasingly clear, however, that a multidisciplinary approach was needed to better integrate service delivery. Multidisciplinary standard setting groups were set up in response to particular concerns. This was a useful way of encouraging professionals to work together in developing understanding of each other's roles, and was to continue to develop as clinical audit came to replace uniprofessional audit as the way forward.

Power

The sort of changes so far described require a significant redistribution of power downwards. The notion of 'bottom up' was one which the PDU was keen to promote. The potential for conflict in an hierarchical organisation is clearly there and cannot be avoided. The shift in the NHS to general management had resulted in an erosion to some extent of traditional power bases. Part of this process involved a devolution of power downwards in an attempt to make those who made decisions about the way in which scarce resources are used more accountable. Thus much effort was made at Seacroft to develop the ward sister role into a ward manager role, with responsibility for ward budgets. This had a knock-on effect, as it became difficult for ward managers to maintain a clinical role also. The F grade nurses (junior sisters) were increasingly seen as needing to have the senior clinical nursing responsibility on the ward, with support from the ward manager. The net effect was to give ward staff much more responsibility than they had previously been used to.

Loyalty

Although staff worked very hard, there was still the typical NHS expectation of a job for life. Resource pressures and the exposure of health services to competition through the internal market meant that such guarantees could no longer be made. The loyalty of staff to the NHS needed to become more focused on the team in which they worked, with a much greater emphasis on the importance of the outcomes of team performance.

Anger

Inevitably perhaps there was considerable anger amongst some about the move to Seacroft. It was important that this was chan-nelled into something creative rather than disruptive, and that meant bringing things out into the open. Staff were not discouraged from expressing anger in meetings as this was thought to be a neces-sary part of the process of adaptation.

Approachability

There was a desire to get away from the perception that decisions were being made behind closed doors, to one where communication was open and honest and decision making transparent.

Social activities to promote change

The social side of the St George's hospital is also worth mentioning. Staff put a lot of energy into events such as patients' parties and Christ-mas pantomimes. These became more frequent as the closure of the hospital approached. There were numerous ward parties, there was the last garden party, the last Christmas dinner. During this time the team bonding became even stronger. Staff members who may have historically not got along suddenly forgot their differences in getting up onto the dance floor. The next day the positive mood continued and had a marked impact on the delivery of patient care. This infor-mal process of team building complemented the more formal sessions.

PDU leader role

The appointment of a new clinical nurse specialist for the elderly at this time did much to support staff during the preparation for the move. This post was later to evolve into the role of clinical leader of the PDU, one which had the task of supporting multidisciplinary practice development, not just nursing development.

Other factors which assisted the process of change were individual performance reviews and personal objective setting for all staff, and different reward systems to acknowledge achievements. These would include access to study leave and study days, access to networks and recognition of work done.

Training

Much effort was put into training staff to cope with a more acute mix of patients than they had been used to at St George's, which accommodated many patients with continuing care needs. There was also some recognition that St George's staff had skills and experience in care of the elderly which would be of value to staff used to working in more acute, particularly medical, settings. The plan was to integrate with the acute medical service already at Seacroft and to have a non-age-related admissions policy. Even so, many medical patients are older people and it was felt that skills transfer should be a two-way thing. It was also important that St George's staff were encouraged to feel some pride in their work and the idea that they had something to offer to others was one it was important to promote. As well as the development of clinical skills there was also an emphasis upon clinical leadership, on relating practice to an evidence base and on evaluation of practice. Specific programmes included training in resuscitation skills, lifting and handling, care planning and record keeping, and management training for clinical staff. There was also a health care assistant training programme.

Support from Region

There was a lot of support from staff in the Nursing Directorate at the Regional Health Authority in firming up ideas and in preparing the bid for accreditation. Along with other aspiring development units from around the region, there was an invitation to discuss possible ways forward at a conference organised by Region, at which various issues were discussed: should there be a single NDU model for the region or should each provider be encouraged to establish an NDU? Are there other ways to advance practice? If so, how can these be linked to policy? What are the policy and organisational implications of NDUs? What support will NDUs need? How will the work of NDUs be shared? How will the NDUs fit into the current work being undertaken on audit, resource management, quality assurance? What about the links with education?

All of these debates were useful in developing ideas. The NDU model was not the only way forward; practice development could and should be pursued to suit local circumstances. The view was held that practice development had to be linked quite firmly with policy direction and business strategy. Practice development is definitely not an add-on to clinical activity, but is essential to maintaining and improving quality of service. The way to link policy and practice development was to make the latter an integral part of the department business plan. The approach Region took was to ask aspiring NDUs to write their own business plans, as if they were somehow separate from the rest of the service. Whilst this may have been helpful in concentrating minds on the need for careful planning, it ignores the realities. In seeking accreditation from Region, Seacroft PDU produced its own business plan as requested. Later, there was a single plan for the Department of Medicine which included practice development. This was the right way forward.

The implications of development units for the wider organisation are still being realised. There was the obvious issue of dissemination of good practice. The PDU was to be seen as a resource for the Trust, a place where new ideas could be tried out, mistakes made and lessons learned. What became increasingly clear, however, was that dissemination was not just about the products of development work, but about spreading a culture as well. In particular, the issue of how to promote real multidisciplinary working and truly effective team work was one which was to exercise our thinking as the years progressed.

The crucial point was that everything was linked. Audit, resource management, quality assurance, education and training, management, policy and business planning were all part of a complex picture. The need was for a truly holistic integration of all of these so as to realise what everyone was after: a high quality, effective and efficient medical service for patients.

As discussions evolved it was possible to place more substance behind the words. Things were coming together. It was important to avoid just blindly following a fashion without thought for the implications or relevance of what was proposed.

King's Fund, NDUs and the PDU

The PDU joined the King's Fund NDU network as there was interest in bidding for the grants to support NDUs. Having independent scrutiny of the PDU was important as a way of reinforcing the belief that what was being done was 'right'. King's Fund ran an information day to promote their accreditation scheme, which two directors attended. There was some difficulty in persuading them of the value of the PDU approach. The issue for them was very much about promoting nursing as a profession. The same level of importance was not attached to this within the PDU. Here it was felt that nursing should develop within the context in which nurses work – in multidisciplinary teams. The PDU application also included a unit of four wards, not the usual one. The bid was unsuccessful in achieving King's Fund Accreditation, and this was no real surprise.

The value of accreditation

It was very encouraging to achieve accreditation from Region in 1993. It had been a long haul. The PDU had been in existence for over a year before being formally acknowledged as such. What was especially gratifying was to have independent scrutiny of everyone's efforts. The accreditation team had been successfully persuaded of the value and relevance of a multidisciplinary approach to practice development. They, to their credit, had responded positively to the arguments that a PDU need not be led by a nurse, could quite successfully develop multidisciplinary practice, and could exist in a four-ward unit. The advantages of accreditation were the opportunities it gave for networking, dissemination and support. It also added credibility to the work and was a way of proving the worth of everyone's efforts in the PDU.

The role of senior management

The support from the senior management was crucial both as a morale booster for the staff and to enable some of the changes proposed. The unit general manager supported the PDU philosophy and actually helped by his non-interventionist style.

Measuring change

In the early 1990s all professions were learning how to deal with the issue of defining and measuring quality. Usually there was a uniprofessional approach, with tools such as the Monitor Index of Nursing Quality (Goldstone et al., 1984) on the market. It was important to demonstrate that change had taken place, not only in organisational and team culture, but in quality of care. As well as auditing multidisciplinary standards, Monitor was used, although its nursing focus

was a little restrictive. Elderly care was so much about multidisciplinary team work that two years later the PDU became part of a
project to develop a multidisciplinary version of Monitor called
EQUATE (Heffernan et al., 1995).

Detailed operational data were collected monthly based on the
patient activity and produced as a report on an annual basis. Based
on the outcome of the data an action plan would be set for areas that
needed improving. Clear aims and objectives were set for the PDU
and for each clinical area. These would be based on research and
audit findings and again evaluated on at least an annual basis.

Disseminating good practice

The issue of dissemination is one which exercises the minds of development unit staff all over the country. In the early years of the PDU,
it was clear what was meant by dissemination: it was about sharing
good practice, about spreading innovation. Later, there was a realisation that dissemination was also about spreading the culture of
multidisciplinary practice development. This became clear when
extending the boundaries of the PDU beyond the original four
wards. The challenge was then how to spread the culture.

The first step had been to produce a profile document so that the
objectives and work of the PDU could be explained. This was seen as
a major step forward by the staff as it clarified their vision for all to
see. The document took a lot of time to produce as ownership of the
document was a major priority. Several drafts were produced before
the final one was agreed.

Achieving accreditation led to invitations to present work at
regional conferences, both in the form of poster displays and seminars.
These were significant steps for many staff, some not used to public
speaking or to talking about their work to others. Such opportunities
were invaluable in boosting the confidence of staff, and not just nurses
either. Although conferences were aimed at nurses, in the PDU's usual
style the multidisciplinary team turned up, and shared the responsibility to host the stand and to present their paper. It was also useful to be
able to compare with others' presentations and to monitor their
progress each time they presented. As they became more experienced
at public speaking, the team became more confident.

Presenting at such events helped to promote the PDU concept
and also challenged the view that an NDU was the best way forward.
Visits to the PDU became more and more frequent, as people heard
about what was being done and wanted to see for themselves. This
helped the dissemination process too.

The PDU encouraged staff to seek publication of their work. For some this meant internal publication in newsletters, for others it meant national journals, giving the unit a much wider audience.

All of these dissemination activities were very good at raising morale. Having such a raised profile did much to raise self-esteem and motivate staff.

The pathway to becoming a PDU

There is no one route to becoming a development unit of whatever sort. The PDU experience was born out of specific circumstances unique to it, and while no one else could be expected to do things in exactly the same way, the lessons were very clear: creating a PDU is very hard work, it involves a major commitment from everyone involved and there are good times when all seems to be going well, and terrible times when everything appears to go wrong. What is vital is that everyone learns from the experience. The lessons about managing change, about organisational development, about promoting team work, about involving patients, are invaluable and can be carried forward to any setting. The cliché about keeping sight of your vision is certainly true.

Chapter 2
The Practice Development Unit concept and structure

Steve Page, Debbie Lee and Hugo Mascie-Taylor

The previous chapter described the early development of the PDU and sought to analyse the context in which this development took place. The aim of this chapter is to define in more detail the initial concept and underlying philosophy of the PDU which emerged from this process, and the structures and systems created to support these in practice.

Looking back on the development of this model now, six years later, it is apparent that its evolution arose from a happy combination of chance circumstances and design, together with a healthy dose of pragmatism. The unit's directors felt an increasing dissatisfaction with existing health service management structures and the professional and departmental barriers which hindered the organisation's ability to focus care around the needs of the patient. In this environment, the directors were searching for a mechanism which would help them to realise some of the benefits of prevalent ideas on 'quality management' in the multidisciplinary health care setting.

In addition, the imminent closure of St George's Hospital and merger of two units also stimulated them to seek an approach to work which would promote personal development and team cohesion, and which would perpetuate and further develop the existing collaborative multidisciplinary ethos.

The timing of the hospital's closure and service moves and fluidity of the prevailing local health service management structures, together with the emergence of NDUs and a number of other movements within health service management, provided the chance element – the favourable climate which enabled their seeds of ideas to germinate and to flourish. The interaction of all these influences over time led to the formulation of a recognisable, formally defined **PDU model**.

One of the interesting features of this model is that although its emphasis was heavily on the stimulation and support of innovation and change, it did not explicitly recognise that an inherent characteristic of the PDU model itself would be its own continued evolution in response to changing circumstances, introduction of new ideas and development of theory from within. This feature has become more apparent with the passage of time and the benefit of hindsight, and subsequent chapters will seek to demonstrate how the model described in this chapter has been developed and refined.

The PDU concept

The PDU was initially based within four 24 bedded wards in the integrated medical/elderly department. Its team consisted of all staff from the multidisciplinary team with input to the wards (therapists, nurses, doctors, managers, social workers and other clinical and non-clinical professionals), with additional support from a Clinical Leader with a multidisciplinary remit, and from the hospital's Quality Assurance Nurse (see figure 2.1).

In addition to providing care of the highest possible standard for its patients, the concept of the unit was that it should serve as a laboratory and test-bed for innovations in patient care and service delivery and should share knowledge gained from such innovation both with other areas in its own organisation, and with practitioners further afield, in order to promote the development of quality patient care.

In order to achieve this within the context of an ordinary clinical area with no additional dedicated resources, the unit sought to provide an enabling environment which encouraged and supported the participation of all staff in examining and developing practice. Key elements in achieving this goal were:

- the adoption of a supportive management style, which would facilitate decision making at appropriate levels
- vigorous support of personal development of all staff
- routine provision of opportunities for free exchange of ideas between members of the multidisciplinary team within a safe and non-judgemental environment.

The unit drew to it the support of educationalists and other professionals, developing partnerships which would maximise the exposure

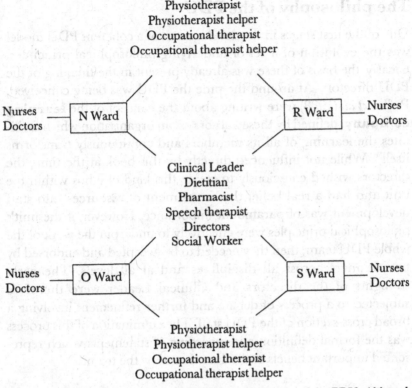

Physiotherapist
Physiotherapist helper
Occupational therapist
Occupational therapist helper

Nurses — N Ward   R Ward — Nurses
Doctors   Doctors

Clinical Leader
Dietitian
Pharmacist
Speech therapist
Directors
Social Worker

Nurses — O Ward   S Ward — Nurses
Doctors   Doctors

Physiotherapist
Physiotherapist helper
Occupational therapist
Occupational therapist helper

Figure 2.1. Initial composition and clinical care setting of the PDU. Although each ward demonstrated its own uniqueness they shared a common philosophy and standards in patient care, strengthening the potential for research and development. The four wards provided a credible test-bed for the multidisciplinary team's research and development. They also provided the platform for the creation of a theoretical framework for practice and allowed the provision of economies of scale.

of its staff to new ideas and relevant expertise, as well as focusing such expertise to a far greater degree than was normally the case, on the clinical practice setting.

The PDU is not necessarily different from other clinical areas in terms of the type of care it delivers, nor does it necessarily develop practice or initiate projects unheard of in any other department. The difference between the PDU and other clinical areas is rather the degree of emphasis on quality of care and its continuous improvement, and the extent to which the fostering of a culture and working environment which supports this is embedded in the structures and everyday management of the unit. Development, evaluation and dissemination of practice are seen as integral to the function of the unit and to the roles of its staff, rather than as extras which are potentially useful once the real work is completed.

The philosophy of the PDU

One of the first stages in the development of a coherent PDU model was the evolution of a set of underlying philosophical principles. Clearly, the basis of these was already present in the thinking of the PDU directors. At around the time the PDU was being conceived, Pedler *et al.* (1988) were writing about the concept of the **learning company**, defined by these authors as 'an organisation which facilitates the learning of all its members and continuously transforms itself'. While not influenced directly by this book at the time, the directors wished consciously to create this kind of ethos within the unit and had a real belief that investment of resources into staff development was of paramount importance. However, if the unit's philosophical principles were effectively to underpin the work of the whole PDU team, then they needed to be accepted and endorsed by practitioners across all disciplines and at all levels. The early thoughts of the directors and Clinical Leader were therefore subjected to a process of debate and further refinement involving a broad cross-section of the PDU staff. The culmination of this process was the formal definition and recording of statements which represented important beliefs and values shared by the team:

- We believe that patients have the right to be involved in decisions about their care and that we should work towards empowering them fully.
- We value the contribution of all members of the multidisciplinary team in promoting high quality care and practice development.
- The PDU is a centre for innovative, creative practice where change for the better is accepted as an essential feature.
- We wish to promote a questioning attitude to all aspects of practice and recognise that there is a need to accept well-considered risk taking as part of development.
- We encourage research-based practice and support its development through education and clinically based research projects.
- We recognise that the PDU has a wider responsibility to encourage and support development in the hospital as a whole.
- We believe that success depends on positive results which benefit patients.

While not necessarily achieving the coherence or comprehensiveness of a complete 'model', these statements of belief by the team were the first real product which sought to define the unit.

These statements, and the degree to which the team 'owned' them, provided the platform for more formal definition of the PDU concept, its aims and its approach to work.

Essential components of the PDU

To some extent many of the elements of PDU philosophy and emerging features of the unit were already enshrined in the concept of the Nursing Development Unit (NDU), which was a clear influence on the PDU, particularly in its early stages. However, in addition to some basic practical differences, the PDU represented a radical departure from the NDU in the extent to which it also accommodated management theory on quality improvement and (related to this and most importantly) in its sharply multi rather than unidisciplinary focus.

The power and potentially negative influence of professional groups on quality and efficiency of patient care had been discussed in the 1970s by authors such as Freidson and Illich. Since then, the emphasis on interprofessional collaboration had been steadily growing within the health service, and this emphasis continues to gain impetus with the more recent focus on clinical effectiveness and evidence-based practice. This, combined with the import of quality management theory into the NHS, which demanded a shift of focus away from the interventions of individual professions or departments in isolation and towards the patient and the process of care in total, caused the managers of the unit to feel a profound dissatisfaction with the status quo.

The prevailing conditions and rationale for change underpinning the emergence of the PDU as a distinct form are illustrated in Figures 2.2–2.8. The bars on each figure can be taken to represent one profession or department within the service. Thus, in Figure 2.2, a number of departments exist, each a different size and shape, probably managed separately and working to a high standard within its own confines.

In Figure 2.3, the line represents the patient's progress through the system. During an average episode of treatment, the patient is likely to come into contact with several professional groups and visit a variety of departments. An ideal progress through this complex system would be represented by a straight line as in Figure 2.3, where each department and professional carried out their assigned role and where, moreover, each interfaced with the other 'seamlessly'.

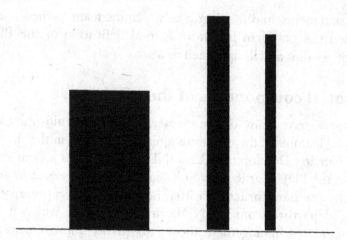

Figure 2.2. A number of departments, each a different size and shape.

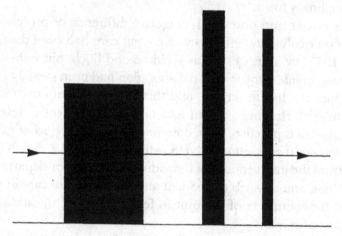

Figure 2.3. The patient's progress through the system: the ideal situation.

However, the reality of the situation is far more accurately represented in Figure 2.4. Here, the zig-zag pattern of the line represents the uneven progress of the patient between professions or departments. Although each individual element of the service may have functioned to the highest standard and may have fulfilled its own role within the system, the patient encounters blockages to progress and inefficiencies at the interfaces between these elements.

The natural inclination for any manager is to wish to remove these blockages by implementing change. However, this is less straightforward than might at first appear. Figure 2.5 illustrates the effect of attempting to introduce such a change in a 'top-down' manner, without seeking to influence the overall culture of the organisation. Instead of reducing the interference in the system and

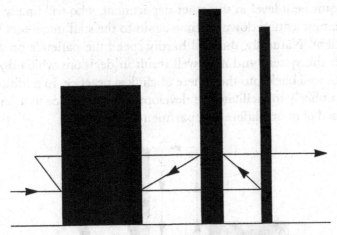

Figure 2.4. The patient's progress through the system: the real situation.

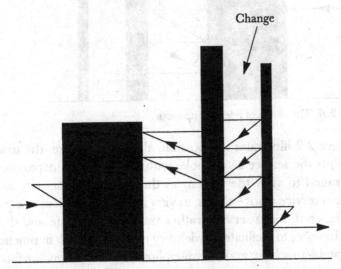

Figure 2.5. Attempting to introduce 'top-down' change.

smoothing the patient's progress at the interfaces between departments, the change is likely to increase these effects, as each department or professional group seeks to compensate and readjust in order to continue to achieve its own targets.

A further effect of the prevailing health service organisation noted by the directors is illustrated in Figure 2.6. When a problem arises in the interface between one group or another, the hierarchical system in place within each does not tend to facilitate an early resolution. Rather, the matter tends to be referred upwards within each department, to the point where a designated person has the authority to make a decision. This will then be communicated to the person at an equivalent level in the other department, who will finally pass this communication down the line again to the staff in contact with the patient. Naturally, this will hardly speed the patient's progress through the system and may well result in decisions which do not translate well back into the sphere of clinical practice. In addition, it will be unlikely to facilitate the development of practice in a service composed of many different departments.

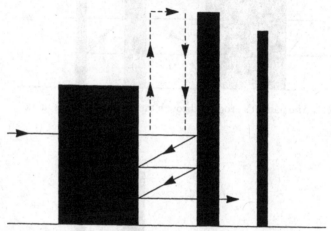

Figure 2.6. The effects of referring upwards.

Figure 2.7 illustrates the possible alternative. Here, the triangle represents the service as a whole, within which each department is encouraged to view the patient as the focus of its activity and to develop a service ethos – that is, to view its own function as one part of a whole, continuous service, rather than as a separate and distinct entity. In order to facilitate the delivery of this approach in practice, to foster problem solving and interdisciplinary collaboration, the function of the organisation's management represented by the small triangle at the top of the diagram, is to create and maintain a culture which will support this process and to ensure that staff closer to the patient are empowered to make decisions and to influence practice. This empowerment of those in direct contact with the patient helps to ensure that changes in practice relate to real patient need and that they are owned and understood by the practitioners who have to implement them.

Figure 2.8 illustrates the ideal scenario, with staff within departments and professions functioning effectively within their own confines, and also in the interfaces between one another. A collaborative, patient-focused culture exists where staff are empowered to take decisions, to resolve problems and to innovate in practice. The result is a smooth progress for the patient through the system and a trouble-free experience.

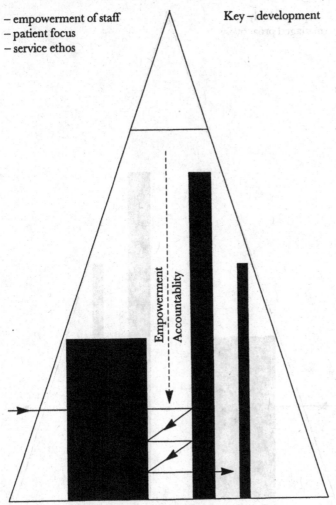

Figure 2.7. A more patient-centred approach.

These diagrams could represent an organisation of any scale, and indeed many of the principles they illustrate were simultaneously being applied across the whole of the PDU's hospital. However, they also illustrate very effectively both the central importance of empowerment in the PDU, and the multidisciplinary basis which differentiates it so markedly from the NDUs which had preceded it.

It is important to acknowledge the contribution of the NDU movement to the philosophical underpinning of the PDU, and undoubtedly the nursing members of the team were initially energised at least in part by their awareness of the NDU movement. However, the divergent concepts outlined above, together with the statement of philosophical principles shared by the whole multidisciplinary team, inevitably led to the definition of the PDU as something quite distinct.

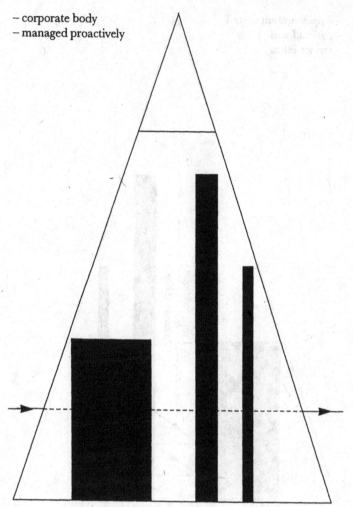

– corporate body
– managed proactively

Figure 2.8. The ideal situation.

The model of the PDU which emerged from subsequent debates within the team was characterised by six essential components. These components informed the specific aims and objectives of the unit and its practical agenda. Similarly, the structures and systems of the PDU were established in order to ensure that these essential elements could be supported. These aims and objectives and the supporting structures and systems implemented in the PDU at its outset will be discussed later in this chapter, although it is important to recognise that these are not fixed, but rather need to vary over time in response to changing clinical priorities and external circumstances. The six essential components, in contrast, have remained consistent over time and are perhaps the only permanent feature of the PDU model. The six components defined by the original PDU team were:

- multidisciplinary teamwork and innovation
- research
- staff empowerment
- patient empowerment
- networking
- dissemination.

Multidisciplinary teamwork and innovation

Within the PDU no one profession takes overall responsibility for leadership of practice or its development. Emphasis is placed on the benefits of sharing expertise and knowledge across professional boundaries in the pursuit of excellence and seamlessness in patient care. Innovation and creativity are encouraged, and a view of change as the norm rather than as something to be feared and avoided is fostered. West (1990) described four features of a culture which would tend to support innovation in the workplace, as follows:

- vision
- participative safety
- climate for excellence
- norms and support for innovation.

The design of the PDU's structures and support systems was aimed as far as possible at promoting and sustaining such a culture across the whole multidisciplinary team. Clinical practice and management arrangements, routine communication, and developmental project work similarly crossed disciplines as appropriate rather than being pursued within each discipline separately.

Research

Research and research-based practice were felt to be integral to the PDU. At a basic level, this meant ensuring that staff from all professional backgrounds were encouraged to question their practice and the practice of the team. Beyond this, a considerable emphasis was placed on the development of skills in critical appraisal and use of research literature in practice. A particularly important consideration in this area was the need to develop such skills across the whole range of professions, where traditionally or because of local development, each individual profession tended to possess very different levels of skill and to employ these to different extents in everyday practice. Different professions also tend to view the value of research or of different forms of research very differently, and in order to promote collaboration it was important to foster a shared understanding of the value of the different research paradigms used by the various professions.

Beyond this, the unit was also felt to exist in order to promote the development of research activity, driven by patient need within the PDU. Much existing research tended to relate to the practice of individual professions, and therefore considerable emphasis was placed on the identification of research subjects related to multiprofessional practice and on the development of multidisciplinary projects to address these.

As with the promotion of multidisciplinary innovation, new structures needed to be created within the unit in order to stimulate and support these processes.

Staff empowerment

The culture of the unit attempted to create an environment where staff of all grades and disciplines could be actively involved in debates and decision-making processes. Enormous emphasis was placed on development of all staff, in order to equip them to participate effectively in the unit's debates and developments. Emphasis was given in this process to work-based approaches to learning, which focused on real practice issues and embedded learning processes within the everyday activity of the unit, rather than approaching development as an expensive add-on activity. Project-based learning was therefore the norm, supported by learning contracts and mentorship arrangements. Reflection on practice by individuals and as a team exercise was built into everyday routine and a culture fostered where staff could openly share their experiences about what had gone well and what could be improved further. Management and leadership functions were designed to be facilitatory, to cross disciplinary boundaries, and to reduce perceptions of superiority of one profession over another. Finally, as a principle, power was delegated downwards within the unit, and wherever possible decision making was shifted as close to the clinical situation as possible.

Patient empowerment

The team believed very strongly in the need to empower patients and their families by encouraging greater participation in decision making about their care. This involved a radical shift of emphasis away from consideration of the professional as the focal point for the service and as the best judge of what was right, and towards an acceptance of the patient as the focus. This demanded a far greater emphasis on health education and provision of information, on accessibility of professional records and on provision of opportunities for patients to express their views of the service and to communicate their priorities.

Networking

The health service environment at the time of the PDU's inception did not tend to encourage sharing of ideas between organisations or disciplines, or collaboration between them in order to develop practice. In some ways this has become more difficult still, particularly on a local level, with the advent of competing NHS trusts. Such activity did take place, but this was largely in spite of the system rather than because of it. In order to foster interdisciplinary and cross-organisational understanding and collaboration, to maximise opportunities for staff development, and to concentrate expert resources within the PDU setting, networking was felt to be an essential component of the unit's approach. This involved, for example, networking between professional groups within the organisation itself, between clinical and academic professionals and between clinical professionals of different organisations. This activity was legitimised within the context of the PDU and promoted as integral to its approach to staff development, rather than seen to be a luxury of no great practical value available only for the elite few, as was previously the case.

Dissemination

An essential part of the PDU's *raison d'être* was felt to be its role as a resource for ideas and information both within the organisation and more widely. Implementation of this role necessitated the development of a far more outward looking organisation than was normally the case. As with networking, it also required the legitimisation of such activity as an integral part of everyday practice, as opposed to the prevailing view of it as an optional extra essentially unrelated to the unit's real work.

Part II of the book devotes a chapter to each of these essential components, drawing out the practical issues encountered in their implementation and seeking to illustrate them by reference to specific developments and project work within the unit.

The structures and systems of the PDU

As stated earlier, the philosophical principles described by the PDU team and the unit's essential components formed its foundation. But simple statements of principles or of desired characteristics, however strongly felt, will not in themselves bring about the desired change. In order to achieve this, it is necessary to actively change existing structures and systems from ones which support the maintenance of the status quo to those which will foster the implementation of the new approach in practice. Such new structures and systems need to be robust and to be integral to the operational function of the unit, if the implementation of the new approach is to be truly rooted in practice, as opposed to being a superficial overlay on top of existing structures and activity.

Within the PDU these practical changes encompassed:

- management structures and style
- organisation of clinical services
- development of clinical leadership and support
- establishment of formal links with educationalists beyond the usual student mentorship arrangements
- creation of a focus on project activity as a practical vehicle for development work.

Each of these is discussed in more detail below, in order to demonstrate how it affected the unit in practice.

Management structures and style

The management arrangements of the PDU were established to reflect the needs of the patient, rather than traditional professional hierarchies and structures. The organisation of the hospital structure into clinical directorates facilitated this process. The PDU was part of the directorate of medicine, and the two PDU directors were the Clinical Director and General Manager of this directorate. This gave the PDU a considerable degree of autonomy from the hierarchy of the hospital as a whole and enabled the development of structures and working patterns which reflected local clinical need. One of the most fundamental changes in this respect involved the inclusion of the management of all of the main clinical professions within the remit of the unit's managers. For example, this meant that nurses were not accountable separately to a nurse manager, or therapists to a therapy manager. This effectively reduced the influence of conflicting managerial or professional forces, while the PDU ethos as a whole ensured that members of the less numerous professions such as the therapies, did not become professionally isolated.

Consultants were also integrated into the organisation more effectively, by attaching them to a particular ward. This fostered greater teamwork between medical and other staff and reduced that sense of consultants as somehow above and beyond the management of the unit which can be so divisive in practice.

Within the unit, managerial accountability was devolved as near to the patient as possible. In particular, this involved the development of the managerial role of the ward sister/charge nurse (taking place as part of a simultaneous hospital-wide initiative). Within the wards, this development of the ward sister role was subsequently reflected and complemented by the parallel development of the role of deputy sisters as leaders of clinical development within the ward and of primary nursing as the preferred mode of care delivery.

Management communication was re-organised in order to reinforce the multiprofessional ethos. Business planning was conducted openly, in order to engage staff of all disciplines and in order to remove some of its attendant mystique. Departmental 'time-outs' were held on a regular basis, and involved a diagonal slice of staff of all disciplines, in order to provide opportunity for discussion of departmental issues and concerns, and for articulation of shared aims and objectives. Open meetings with staff were organised on a routine basis, particularly where major developments were taking place, in order to ensure that all staff felt involved in the process. Similarly, as well as the regular management meetings where the business of the unit was conducted, weekly information meetings were held which were open to any member of staff within the unit. The functions of these meetings were to:

- brief staff regarding any changes
- discuss operational issues
- consider developments within the PDU
- enable leaders of project groups to obtain and disseminate information on their respective activity to all staff.

These arrangements did not preclude the formation of other staff groups or the meeting of *ad hoc* groups, either to aid communication, to provide mutual support or to promote specific developments. The intention was to create an open and supportive environment with free flowing horizontal and vertical communication, which would ensure that the whole workforce was well informed and engaged in the process, and would stimulate the development of new ideas.

The use of these forums to agree shared aims and objectives enabled the unit to arrive at a clear programme of development. From the outset, these agreed programmes were clearly defined in the form of PDU action plans. These plans were available to all staff within the unit and provided a valuable means of establishing the shared sense of direction within the unit's team. The implementation of individual performance review and personal development planning for staff within the unit facilitated the discussion of each individual's role within the larger picture as well as helping to focus their development in areas which would promote the unit's ethos.

These measures in total were aimed at enabling staff to work with maximum autonomy and with a positive belief in their ability to influence the quality and efficiency of the service they provided, and in so doing to minimise the confusion, frustration and conflict characteristic of many traditional health service organisations, key outcomes of which tend to be stasis and maintenance of the status quo.

Organisation of clinical services

Clinical services were also restructured, in order to reflect the 'patient focused' ethos of the unit. The integration of acute medical and elderly services within the department of which the PDU was part demonstrated a commitment to the principle of services defined by patients' needs rather than by traditional structures. This also facilitated a sharing of resources and cross-fertilisation between teams of practitioners with historically different skills and perspectives on patient care.

The organisation of the PDU around four wards, rather than just one, also facilitated this process. At around the time the PDU was beginning to emerge, literature was starting to appear on the 'patient focused hospital' concept (for example, Lathrop *et al.*, 1991). This literature supported views within the PDU that hospitals tended to be organised around departments and individual professions rather than around the needs of the patient, and that this adversely affected quality and efficiency of care. The patient focused hospital concept is built on five main principles:

- the need to streamline documentation systems
- movement of routine services closer to the patient, rather than locating them in distant departments, as is the norm

- broadening the skills of care-givers – what is commonly known as 'multiskilling'
- simplification of processes
- focusing the patient population within individual wards, so that patients with as similar needs as possible are cared for in the same place (adapted from Lathrop *et al.*, 1991).

Although the PDU did not aim to pursue the patient focused hospital concept in its entirety, and added its own flavour to the concept in its emphasis on patient and carer empowerment and involvement, some of these principles were certainly in the minds of the PDU's leaders.

The importance of the changes to records systems to the PDU's early development are discussed in a later chapter, and other chapters will examine in detail some of the ways in which the PDU helped to challenge and simplify existing health care processes. The second principle, of moving services closer to the patient, was a key feature of the way in which the services within the PDU were established from the outset. As indicated earlier, the consultants worked to specific wards, rather than functioning as roving professionals separated from everyday patient care. Similarly, named therapists, dietitian, pharmacist and social worker were clearly identified as part of the PDU team. Furthermore, therapy services were also moved into a location adjacent to the PDU wards themselves, and away from their original central department. Physiotherapy and occupational therapy assessment and treatment therefore took place immediately next door to the wards. At a later stage, this movement of services closer to the patients was developed further, with the delivery of cardiac rehabilitation classes within the unit, and the relocation of cardiology services to a location next to the wards. This facilitated communication and teamworking between the professions in the care of individual patients and also reduced the amount of travelling time and portering for patients between wards and departments.

It also promoted the sharing of skills between professions – for example between physiotherapists and nurses – even though this aspect was not explored on a formal basis.

These developments were not without their problems, of course. For example on a practical level, while facilitating treatment of in-patients, the lack of a centralised department for therapies initially created difficulties in treatment of out-patients, who could often be found wandering around the medical block searching for the appropriate treatment room. This problem was soon overcome, however, with improved directions and signposting. Ultimately, however, it is our belief that the physical proximity of the majority of the multidisciplinary care taking place within the PDU's wards, inevitably supported the development of trust, effective communication and teamworking across the whole team, with significant benefits for the unit's patients.

Clinical leadership and support

The role of Clinical Leader within the PDU initially evolved from the Clinical Nurse Specialist post already in existence. Before the transition to Clinical Leader, the role was focused on the development of nursing and nurses, and even though there were examples of effective collaboration between professions, the traditional demarcation between them was broadly maintained. In the PDU context, however, the role was clearly defined as one of leadership of clinical development across the whole multidisciplinary team. The person fulfilling this role could not hope to be a clinical expert in all areas within her/his remit in the way a clinical nurse specialist or senior therapist can be. This therefore necessitated a further development of the role away from pure clinical expertise and towards breadth of vision and skills of facilitation, coordination, motivation and management of change. The aims of the role were to empower and encourage staff from all professions to function as knowledgeable, reflective and autonomous practitioners who work together in harmony, and galvanisation of the different elements of the team towards defining and achieving shared goals. In the early stages, the Clinical Leader concentrated heavily on clinical practice within the PDU, working very closely with individuals and groups of staff and often working directly with patients on one or other of the wards. This emphasis was perhaps a feature of the post's original nursing emphasis, but was also a key element of the success of the unit in its early stages as it ensured that its work was energised and driven at grass-roots level. As the unit has matured, as ward and department leaders have themselves become more empowered and as the context in which the PDU functions has become steadily more politically charged, the emphasis has gradually shifted away from direct care and day-to-day contact on the wards.

The Clinical Leader also developed over time as a key link between the clinical team and the managers of the PDU, ensuring that work on management, clinical and professional issues was well integrated. Initially the influence of the newly evolved Clinical Leader role on the development of the unit was relatively low.

However, very rapidly the role developed into an essential catalyst and driving force, ensuring the high profile of clinical priorities in the subsequent evolution of the unit and its business plans.

The Clinical Leader's responsibilities as originally defined in the PDU included:

- leadership, coordination and evaluation of practice in the unit
- fostering an educational climate tailored to suit individual needs within an interdisciplinary framework
- guidance of staff towards development designed to empower both practitioners and patients
- preparation of proposals and identification of resources to develop practice, and seeking external resources to support this process where appropriate
- creation and maintenance of links with outside agencies – for example, university departments, other hospitals, community services
- liaison with the PDU directors in business and strategic planning and to facilitate developments
- dissemination of PDU information – for example, through conferences, education programmes and clinical groups.

The role initially evolved from an existing post, rather than being created entirely from scratch and was quite unlike anything any of the practitioners within the unit had experienced before. Because of this, there was a need to develop and refine it in practice and this meant that the shift away from a primarily nursing emphasis towards full multidisciplinary leadership was gradual rather than instantaneous. This evolution was further complicated by the fact that perceptions of the original postholder were inevitably coloured by her original nursing remit. Cross-discipline frictions and misunderstandings certainly arose at times because of this. However, the tangible benefits of the role in facilitating and coordinating work across a number of disciplines, while clearly recognising the unique contribution of each, became apparent in specific clinical project work, and it gradually grew to be well-established and valued by all disciplines. It became recognised that while the postholder was herself a nurse, the specific professional qualification was less important than the broader leadership and facilitatory skills, and that potentially in the future the role could be fulfilled by a member of any profession. (The further development of the leader role as the PDU continued to mature is discussed in Chapter 3.)

In addition to identified senior professionals within each discipline, the Clinical Leader drew further support from a nurse with a hospital-wide quality assurance remit. While not entirely dedicated to the PDU, this person played a key part in complementing the clinical focus of the leader with quality, audit and research-related skills and supported the development of academic rigour in evaluation of PDU work. This role itself was in an evolutionary state throughout the early development of the PDU and was only crystallised at a much later stage as the unit's Research Practitioner. In spite of its significant contribution, it could not be said, therefore, to be a clear part of the initial 'PDU model'. (Again, this development is discussed in greater detail in the next chapter.)

In order to support the leadership of the unit, two formal groups were established – the PDU Steering Group and the Research Advisory Group (RAG). The former was established as the main umbrella of support for the unit and consisted of individuals who were considered to be either a specialists in a relevant field which would complement the PDU's own expertise, or who had enough power and influence in the external environment to advise the PDU on its developments. A further influencing factor was the level of personal ability and motivation observed in the individual. The group was established with the following terms of reference:

- to monitor the achievement of the PDU's aims and objectives
- to support and advise on current and future developments
- to publicise PDU activity.

The precise membership naturally changed over time for a variety of reasons, but at various times included:

- PDU directors
- clinical leader
- hospital general manager
- hospital head of professional development
- director of clinical support services (manager of therapies and other 'professions allied to medicine')
- manager of community rehabilitation services
- head of pharmacy department
- consultant physician
- principal university lecturer.

On reflection, it might also have been useful to include a representative of purchasers on this group, although when it was established the NHS reforms were at a relatively early stage. Also, a representative of users of the service could also have been included in order to further promote the unit's aims with regard to patient empowerment.

The RAG was established in order to further the objectives of the PDU with regard to the development of a multidisciplinary research culture. Its functions were to:

- provide advice and encouragement to all staff wishing to carry out research
- provide expert advice on development and implementation of specific research projects
- support staff in the publication of research
- offer a multidisciplinary perspective on research activity
- review progress against the PDU's research-related objectives.

These meetings ran once each month and staff of all disciplines and at any level were encouraged to attend, to discuss their ideas or work. This brought directly to the clinical staff of the unit an unusually high level of academic, clinical and managerial expertise and also helped further to promote the multidisciplinary focus of the unit's work. (The operation of this group and its further development are discussed in detail in Chapter 7.)

The final element of support for the PDU established at the outset as a essential feature of the model, as in the NDU approach, was the close partnership with educators. The contribution of academic professionals to the PDU is multifaceted and ranges from promoting an awareness of theoretical trends and consideration of their practical applications, to assistance on an individual or group level with staff development and the implementation of educationally sound teaching and learning within the unit.

Within the PDU approach they may be collaborators on individual projects or, as described above, members of more formal advisory groups. In addition, their contribution tends to promote the development of a questioning attitude among staff and of confidence in practitioners who may not previously have felt able to undertake formal academic study and may therefore have had little exposure to such thinking. It serves also to support the PDU's goal of embedding development within its everyday work.

In order to facilitate this input, the unit sought to create semiformal partnerships with named individuals from higher education as well as to promote further collaborations on an *ad hoc* basis as appropriate to support specific pieces of work. The more formal liaisons enabled the unit to develop the role of educators as an integral part of the team rather than simply as visitors and helped to ensure mutual understanding and continuity of development over long periods.

Project focus of the PDU

In its early stages the PDU focused on a relatively small number of key projects, and this was probably essential to the unit's success. These projects were carefully selected to promote the development of the 'empowerment' culture within the unit – for example, development of the ward sister role and of primary nursing, implementation of resource management tools within the wards; or to support the growth of interdisciplinary collaboration – for example, development of multidisciplinary records, definition and audit of multidisciplinary standards, nutrition audit and self-medication pilot.

Within the early multidisciplinary project groups established within the unit a structured approach to problem solving was encouraged, which broadly followed the following steps:

- **Identification of the problem**: raising of an issue through one of the communication forums set up within the PDU or through informal routes.
- **Expression of the problem**: examination and more precise definition of the issue through debate within the multidisciplinary team.
- **Ownership of the problem**: identification of appropriate individuals to lead and participate in tackling the problem, based on their personal interest, professional involvement and skills.
- **Formation of goals**: Agreement of a vision of where the team would like to be with regard to the specific problem. In addition to discussion within the various PDU groups, other means commonly used to inform this process would include use of questionnaires, focus group discussions, literature reviews, and networking with other units.
- **Comparison of the current situation with the agreed vision or goals**: Identification of deficits and of aspects needing further investigation and groundwork before specific changes could be agreed – for example, via more comprehensive review of literature.

- **Selection and planning of desirable and feasible changes**: in addition to the issues intrinsic to the problem itself, the project group also need to consider whether their objectives will be consistent with the goals of the unit as a whole. The planning process would also include consideration of resource implications, timescales, key stakeholders in any change and ultimate dissemination of the work.
- **Action:** usually, initial stages of any action involved a pilot phase, where processes could be tested and refined prior to commencement of larger scale work or changes involving the unit as a whole.
- **Evaluation:** a written summary evaluation of the project as a whole, including any issues in its implementation.
- **Dissemination:** sharing of results and lessons learned during implementation with others, either within the hospital or beyond, and celebration of achievements by individuals involved.

This project-oriented approach enabled the rapid development of specific areas of work and production of early successes which were important to the belief in the unit both from within and from those outside. The structured approach, facilitated by the Clinical Leader and other senior staff, was also an important mechanism for the development of skills within the PDU team. In its more mature state it is not possible to define the PDU in terms simply of the project work it undertakes. In doing so there could be a danger of promoting a relatively narrow, short-term view and preventing a longer-term development of strategically planned programmes of activity. Nevertheless, a focus on project activity remains an important feature of the unit, as a means of engaging and developing individuals, of reinforcing the multidisciplinary ethos, and finally of helping to ensure that the unit does not exist merely for the purposes of its own continuation, but to develop practice in priority areas.

Conclusion

It was argued earlier that the PDU is a service model designed to make the patient the focus of hospital activity and attempts were made to draw out some of the similarities between the PDU approach and the American 'patient focused hospital' concept, which was widely debated in the management literature of the early 1990s. Another related strand of management literature emerging concurrently with the early development of the PDU, was that discussing **process re-engineering**. It was Michael Hammer (1990) who first coined the phrase **business re-engineering** although the concept had been around for at least 20 years. This is broadly an approach to analysing the way in which organisations deliver their service and identification of opportunities for radically improving this service by simplification of the organisation's processes and supporting systems.

Within the re-engineering approach the primary focus is the design and implementation of cross-functional processes which ignore traditional organisational demarcations. Hammer and Champney (1993) identified six principles characterising the process, which relate well to some of principles underlying the PDU:

- organise around outcomes not tasks
- have those who use the output of the process perform the process
- subsume information processing work into real work that produces the information
- treat geographically dispersed resources as though they were centralised
- link parallel activities instead of integrating their tasks
- put the decision point where the work is performed and build control into the process.

Clearly some of this literature has emerged since the initial development of the PDU and there is no suggestion therefore that there was originally a conscious decision on the part of the unit's leaders at the outset to employ process re-engineering within the PDU. However, even though it was not formally used at the time, this term characterises well the process initiated within the unit, and the PDU itself can reasonably be viewed as an outcome of a form of re-engineering. As the unit continued to develop, its leaders' awareness of this literature increased and it was used more explicitly to inform the development of the PDU and to illustrate its modes of working.

Within many re-engineering programmes the initial attention tended to be on 'hard issues' like the processes and systems; 'soft issues' like the people of the organisation, their values, skills and behaviour were often considered as being of secondary importance. Within the process undertaken in the development of the PDU equal, if not greater, attention was also paid to these soft issues, in recognition of the fact that these issues had at least as powerful an effect on the quality and efficiency of the unit's processes as the design of the processes themselves.

After the first year of its development, the PDU model was becoming established. A substantial re-engineering process had been undertaken, with some success in terms of change both to work processes and structures within the multidisciplinary team, and to the underlying culture, skills and vision of the team which informed these processes. An attempt, at least partly successful, had been made to start with the proverbial blank sheet of paper in the planning of the unit, which was greatly facilitated by the need to establish a new service after the closure of the old hospital. As noted in the previous chapter, not all staff adapted well into this new environment. However, by the end of the first year, the majority of staff were committed to and enthused by the new work environment. Real changes to this work environment were evident in day-to-day practice and the unit was able to point to a range of concrete practical achievements against its initial project objectives. (Table 2.1 presents a summary of some of these practical achievements, in order to give a flavour of the unit's early activity.) The unit was beginning to develop a reputation as a desirable place to work and its early achievements at all levels offered the team the chance to celebrate successes. This was in itself a key component in the reinforcement of the team spirit and ethos of the unit.

Particularly in the early stages of development, the unit was moving at a significantly faster pace than the organisation around it. The structures and systems set down by the wider organisation could become barriers to the PDU's goals of continuous learning and development of practice and could cut across the unit's multidisciplinary ethos. There was a natural tendency, therefore, to throw the rule book out of the window in the early stages. Frequently, this challenge to the prevailing system was a healthy phenomenon, if distinctly uncomfortable for the organisation as a whole. However, at times the strong leadership and support from the steering group was necessary, in order to point out to the team that some of the rules were there for their protection rather than simply for the purposes of perpetuating management bureaucracy.

Finally, we should add a note of caution to this discussion. On a practical level, in spite of the unit's advances, small frictions could still sometimes arise where the needs of patient care in the unit and traditional professional requirements or ways of working were in conflict with one another. Some professional practices and viewpoints remained difficult to shift and in order not to alienate sections of the team from the entire PDU process it was necessary to focus on areas where there was positive agreement and to work around the

Table 2.1 Practical achievements of the PDU in the first year

PDU aim	Achievements
To provide high quality, effective care for all patients	Initiation of multidisciplinary standard setting and audit against these standards
	Introduction of clinical objectives for each ward
	Routine audit of patient accidents and pressure sores
	Implementation of GRASP workload measurement tool to wards
To encourage new approaches to patient care	Initiation of critical review of documentation in the multidisciplinary team
	Pilot and evaluation of self-medication programme for older patients
To promote accountability and autonomy in nursing and therapy professions	Development of primary nursing
	Development of multidisciplinary communication
	Development of multidisciplinary peer audit
To develop staff to their full potential	Agreement of personal development plans as part of individual performance review process
	Organisation of in-house PDU education drawing on skills within the team
To support research within the PDU	Education related to research appreciation and use
	Identification of areas for research
	Successful application for small scale project grants
Development of a supportive management style which would involve staff in decision-making processes	Introduction of management training for G-grade nurses and lead therapists and development of sisters, role
	Introduction of multidisciplinary and project planning forums
To introduce methods to evaluate change	Monthly audit of standards and dissemination of results
	Review of progress against clinical objectives
	Agreement of appropriate evaluation of specific project work at its outset
To promote strong links with educational institutions	Membership of King's Fund nursing development network
	Development of close working relationship with local college of health and polytechnic and development of access to relevant programmes

more contentious issues and return to them at a later stage, in order
to tackle them incrementally. Also, it remained the case that while
the majority of staff were motivated and energised by the new developments, there remained a significant minority whose practice was

unaffected by the changes. Changing cultures and work patterns within organisations or professions is a complex and long-term undertaking and the authors would not wish to claim that the PDU model overcame all of these issues in one dramatic movement, nor even that they were all ultimately resolved.

Ultimately, the implementation of the PDU model outlined above provided an atmosphere where such developments could have greatest likelihood of success. They resulted in rapid achievements on many levels and enabled the unit's managers to transform the stressful closure of a well loved but essentially static service into the creation of a wholly new and dynamic unit. The model has not remained unaltered since its original definition, but has subsequently needed to be adapted and further refined, in response to continually changing circumstances. However, the model as defined above represented a strong foundation on which the unit's team could continue to build, and remains the core of what the PDU is all about.

The remainder of the book attempts to explore in more detail how this initial model has been developed and to illustrate each of its key components in action.

Chapter 3
Developing the
model

Steve Page

Pressure and change

In the first two chapters the origins of the PDU and its early development have been discussed in some detail. It is clear from these accounts that the unit did not simply occur at random, but that a number of essential conditions prevailed which enabled it to emerge and which fuelled its early development.

These involved:

- a planned move to a new purpose-built unit
- a sharp focus on skills development and team-building honed by the impending move
- managers and clinicians with a shared vision and commitment to the multidisciplinary approach
- the excitement of developing a new model for multidisciplinary practice within the unit, unique to and owned by the team
- a clear set of goals arising from the move and the emerging model
- a thriving practice development network in the Yorkshire region.

These conditions enabled the unit to develop its agenda rapidly, to achieve notable early successes and to emerge as a leader in multidisciplinary practice development within the region. Plans had been created and implemented by the team, and rewards for their successes were tangible at an early stage. The plans for the hospital as a whole were clear and relatively stable and this provided a solid framework within which staff felt safe to innovate and to challenge the boundaries of their practice.

What happens though, when some of these ideal conditions – both internal and external – begin to shift or to crumble? How are the enthusiasm and commitment of the team retained? How is continuity in the unit's work ensured? How do the unit's plans remain live, vibrant and relevant?

Within 18 months of its original inception these questions began to be raised, and a number of key changes were taking place which exerted a major influence on the unit and to which it needed urgently to be able to adapt.

This chapter describes some of the specific conditions affecting the PDU after its initial phase of intense activity and the early flush of success. It also analyses the continued development of the PDU in response to these conditions, to give a (hopefully) 'warts and all' account of how it survived and continued to grow. In doing this, it is hoped that it will be possible to demonstrate both the vital importance of adaptability to survival and to production of relevant work, and also the fact that this can be achieved within the framework of a flexible model for practice but without compromising the essential tenets of the unit's philosophy.

Pressures and changes on the unit

A period of almost continuous organisational change

In less than two years, the hospital in which the unit is situated had belonged technically to four different organisations. An anticipated merger with the community trust and planned development into a community hospital facility was replaced by an actual merger ultimately with a large teaching hospital trust and consequent sharp refocus on provision of acute services. With this level of organisational change inevitably came a constant shifting of priorities. Staff on the ground were confused about what exactly the hospital expected of them and there was real anxiety at all levels about job security. The shared vision defined as essential by authors on change (West, 1990) was virtually impossible. In fact, the situation appeared to swing between the impression of a total void in terms of vision and a veritable Babel of different visions. Either way, there was little which staff in wards or department could truly believe in, beyond the level of their everyday contact with patients.

Within the PDU, a shared vision continued to exist to a large extent and belief in the unit's philosophy remained strong, particularly among its original team. However, this philosophy and way of working appeared to be at odds with that surrounding the unit. With no clear understanding of how the PDU was to fit into the shifting broader organisation and a consequent lowering of its perceived significance to the hospital came also a reduction in practical support from outside the unit. The impossibility of supporting any 'roll-out' of PDU innovations to other areas in such fluid conditions only exacerbated this, and the PDU was consequently beginning to grow isolated and introspective.

The anxiety about job security not unnaturally dampened enthusiasm for any form of risk taking at all levels. Energy was channelled instead into measures to secure one's own safety, or into job hunting, or simply into the act of worrying itself. Innovation in clinical practice paled into insignificance next to the rumour that the entire medical/elderly service might close.

Changes to personnel

During this period of organisational change, there was also significant turnover of staff within the PDU. During its early development the workforce had been very stable relative to that in the hospital as a whole. The opportunities for personal development and level of interesting activity within the unit had not only been a considerable incentive for staff to remain within the unit, but also proved a major attraction to students and qualified nurses in other areas – functioning in much the same way as described for the US Magnet Hospitals (McLure et al., 1983).

During this unsettled period, however, staff turnover increased, both as a result of a search by many for more secure jobs and of the reduction in satisfaction with what the PDU was able to achieve. In addition to this general increase in turnover, a number of key individuals, all of whom had been involved in the PDU from its origins, moved on to job promotions. Ironically, this reflected the unit's success in developing its staff, although perhaps also the unit's circumstances provided an added incentive at the time.

First to move on was the original PDU Clinical Leader, followed shortly after by the unit's Operational Manager and Clinical Director – in effect the three driving forces behind its original establishment. Following this, two of the unit's three ward sisters also moved on. In all cases the staff were replaced. However, not unnaturally this added to the climate of uncertainty and also created a hiatus in terms of leadership and coordination of practice development during the period in which original members of the team wound down and new members found their feet.

This change in both the unit's leaders and the team as a whole also had major implications for the team's identification with and 'ownership' of the unit's philosophy.

Resource restrictions

As in the health service as a whole, the PDU experienced an increasingly tight rein on resources. It had never been the recipient of additional funding, with the exception of that arising from successful development, audit and research grant bids. However, in the early stages it had been possible to fund some secondment opportunities from within the unit's staffing budget and to support small scale developments from a mixture of the unit budget and a variety of fund-raising schemes. However, the budgetary squeeze reduced this flexibility within the unit's resources and in particular made project or developmental secondments impossible, given the emphasis on merely covering the wards and departments for essential clinical work.

Beyond this, however, resource restrictions effectively killed off one of the PDU's most rigorous, successful and well-publicised pieces of work. A grant-funded project to pilot a self-medication scheme for elderly patients had been implemented after painstaking development work. This had subsequently been evaluated in a research study also funded by external grant, with results clearly demonstrating a benefit to patients in terms of increased knowledge of drugs and compliance with their regime post-discharge. The results were published in journals, conference papers and even on Radio 4. Unfortunately, in order to implement the scheme in practice following the exhaustion of the pilot funding, money was needed to fund additional pharmacy technician time for individual labelling of the patients' drugs. This money could not be found, and therefore after a year and a half of effort and much widely publicised success, the whole scheme had simply to be abandoned.

This episode and the lessons learned from it will be discussed in more detail in the next chapter. However, the impact on the team's confidence and motivation of this failure to assimilate one of the unit's most successful and celebrated projects into practice, can hardly be overstated.

These changes and their sequelae in terms of negative pressures on innovation and meaningful, planned practice development are not unique to Seacroft. Indeed, to the majority of health service trusts such issues are the everyday backdrop to current practice. However, in many organisations – and notably in some of the Nursing Development Units (NDUs) – such pressures have ultimately ridden rough-shod over the development culture and have crushed the fragile innovations in practice.

There is considerable musing over the question of whether the NDU model, for example, is a valid one with a significant impact on practice, and over its many successes and equally apparent weaknesses. A crucial issue overlooked in this debate, however, is the more fundamental question of whether any fixed model will remain valid for very long in the NHS environment of ever-accelerating change. To some extent perhaps the NDU model was defined in too concrete terms too soon – a victim of its own success and high profile – limiting its potential for adaptation and further development.

The PDU was primarily a development in response to local needs and conditions, however. While a model was defined on paper, it was not one which was dependent on the sanction of an external body and therefore there remained significant freedom of movement in terms of adapting and building on the unit's basic principles and modes of work in response to continuing changes going on around it.

This does not mean that the pressures on the unit were shrugged off without pain, nor that they did not severely diminish its capacity for productive work. At times the condition of the unit was dire – at one point its development agenda had virtually ground to a total halt, with morale and self-belief in the team on their death-bed. What it did mean, however, was that recovery even from this desperately low point was possible, and that the unit was able to re-emerge early as a positive force even while the broader organisation around it continued to struggle.

Adaptation and revitalisation

One of the initial strengths of the PDU was the powerful sense of ownership among the team and a truly shared philosophy and vision about where the unit should be going. The leadership and participative processes which brought this about have been described in the preceding chapters. However, membership of a team gradually shifts over time.

The usual approach to dealing with this phenomenon is to induct new staff into the philosophy and approaches of the organisation. The organisation is perceived as something constant, to which the individual is assumed to be either naturally suited or able to adapt. To a degree, this can be accommodated without any detrimental effect, with the result merely that one or two individuals may feel less at ease or engaged than the bulk of the team. Where a significant proportion of the team has changed, however, this assumption can be more dangerous.

Staff will be recruited by the unit's managers at least in part for their ability to think innovatively and for their willingness to challenge received wisdom. Such people are unlikely to enjoy being indoctrinated into the 'right way' of thinking without any opportunity for discussion about what that way might be.

An important and distinguishing feature of the PDU is that, while underpinned by a number of essential principles and definable as a 'model' in the abstract sense (i.e. amenable to the drawing of nice diagrams and pictures), it is not assumed to be static. There is an acceptance that within this broad framework, it will need constantly to develop and adapt to new circumstances, in order to survive and to remain vibrant. The capacity to achieve this is generated by the members of the team themselves.

With this in mind, considerable effort is spent on a regular process of reaffirmation, supported by 'time-out' events and mini-workshops as well as written consultations and the Clinical Forum described below. Such discussions also facilitate a sharing of ideas between old and new staff, thereby helping to prevent the chasm which can often arise between the two groups. Existing staff learn from and are challenged by new members of the team, so that the prevailing ideas are subtly challenged. This therefore enables new staff to participate in redefining the unit's philosophy and aims, resulting in continuous subtle changes to the PDU approach and a belief among the new members of the team that they have a voice in the unit.

This process, following the severe dip in fortunes described at the beginning of this chapter, helped to shift the energy of the PDU team back from negative to positive, so that while the organisation all around it continued to undergo significant change, the PDU – like a lean and well-focused company coming out of a recession – emerged early in this process as a flexible and vibrant unit, with a clearly focused agenda.

During this process, the main principles on which the work of the PDU was based were not radically changed, but were restated in words belonging to the new team. Seven key points were identified, which can be seen to have evolved from the unit's original philosophy. These were that the unit should be:

- patient focused
- multidisciplinary

- empowering of patients and staff of all disciplines and grades to participate as equals in any practice debates or developments
- innovative
- clinically and academically credible
- relevant – to the needs of the patients, the broader organisation and the wider context of health care
- well integrated into the trust within which it is based.

These principles serve to highlight both the similarities and essential differences between the PDU and NDU concepts. For example, with regard to the third principle: although NDUs may undertake multi-disciplinary developments, other disciplines participate as 'guests' of nurses, rather than as equal partners. The fifth and sixth principles are crucial to the PDU approach, but significantly less heavily emphasised in the NDU setting. These issues will be discussed in more detail in Chapter 5.

In terms of practical work undertaken in the unit, a number of legitimate areas for activity were identified by the team:

- work promoting and developing the philosophy and culture of the unit, and development of staff. Attention to these areas was felt to be essential to underpin any other activities.
- Clinically focused practice development, audit and research.
- Work with a professional, organisational and managerial empha-sis, for example, developments in interdisciplinary communica-tion and examination of role boundaries.
- Dissemination of work, both internally within the trust's hospitals and externally.

With the seven principles in mind and a focus on these key areas, the team began to redefine its priorities and to plan developmental work which was both practical and meaningful within its new circumstances. Debate within the unit followed as a natural conse-quence of changes both internal and external. Out of this debate arose a shift in the focus of the multidisciplinary team. A renewed philosophy and objectives were generated by this team, resulting in the development of practical plans for activity which were owned by the team itself.

Finally, these plans and their implementation exerted a powerful effect on the plans of the directorate and hospital as a whole, leading to a significant shift in quality strategy and development of profes-sional practice.

The process can clearly be seen to equate to that described in Pedler, Boydell and Burgoyne (1988) as characteristic of a **learning company**. That is, an organisation where strategy and practice can be seen as a cycle, where one drives the other in equal measure. It illustrates also the principles of empowerment and patient focus in action – empowerment, clearly, because of the extent to which any members of staff were able genuinely to contribute to the organisation's plans, and more unusually, to see their contribution being taken beyond the level of token input, to the point of seeing concrete examples of their ideas being used to shape the organisation's plans.

It is worth commenting at this stage that skills of facilitation and attentive listening are vital to the development of an empowered workforce. However, a commitment by the organisation to act on ideas expressed is what raises the exercise beyond the merely cosmetic level.

The principle of patient focus within the unit is used in the broadest possible sense of being driven by patients' needs and wishes, rather than in the widely-used technical/managerial sense coined in the USA. It is reflected in Figure 3.1.

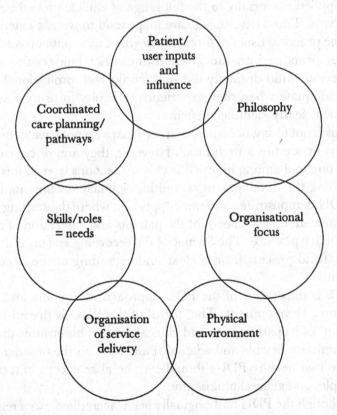

Figure 3.1. Patient focus in the PDU.

The patient focus of the unit ensured that plans were driven by the needs of patients and carers, rather than by managerial or professional hobbyhorses, or by abstract theory.

In many instances in the health service we appear to be searching for some universal panacea to apply to all situations, for example, some aspects of professional models, quality improvement theory, process re-engineering, and at a clinical practice level, the frenzied development of care maps and pathways over recent years.

There is a tendency to identify the solution before the problem and then to force the solution to fit, rather than developing the solution out of the problem itself. The PDU's focus enabled its team to develop approaches which responded directly to specific circumstances and allowed it to remain unencumbered by such limitations, while being free to draw eclectically on theory from whatever source would be useful at the time.

To look at this another way, it could be argued that much health service activity can be seen as a triumph of form over content. The issue of care maps is a classic example, where a format is devised and then applied universally to the full range of clinical procedures and conditions. Those developing care maps tend to wrestle extensively with the practical issues of fitting the needs of their patients and their clinical practice into the given framework. The result can be cumbersome and distinctly user-unfriendly, with professionals feeling inadequate when they experience difficulty in using a system with such clearly identified benefits.

This is not to say, of course, that care maps do not have significant benefits or are not a useful tool. However, they are, of course, just that – one tool among many. The chapter sections later in this book describing the development of multidisciplinary documentation in the PDU demonstrate a different approach, where the starting point is identification of the needs of the patients and carers and of multidisciplinary practice. The format of the recording system is derived as a natural process from a clear understanding of the necessary content.

This is illustrative of the PDU approach as a whole and of its continued development. The 'form' of the PDU is driven by the 'content' of its patient care and clinical work. This ensures that the PDU remains flexible and adaptable and also, on the broader level, that no two healthy PDUs should ever be alike except in terms of principles and general philosophy.

Although the PDU had originally been 'accredited' via a regional scheme for NDUs and PDUs, this realisation led the team to the view that continued accreditation against set criteria could only be inhibiting and would not reflect the continuous development of the unit.

Developments in structure and processes

In the wake of this review, the structure and support mechanisms of the unit also needed to change, to enable it to deliver its objectives effectively.

The clinical leader role itself was one of the first areas of significant change. This post originated in the Clinical Nurse Specialist role and in the early stages, while moving to a more multidisciplinary rather than purely nursing focus, bore many of the hallmarks of such roles. The leader was focused sharply on the clinical areas, spending a large proportion of time within the unit's boundaries and spending some shifts each week working on the wards. Dissemination of PDU work outside the unit was also a key part of the role. At the outset, while there was some need for the leader to become involved in the organisational politics surrounding the unit, this was a relatively slight commitment as the bulk of this activity was undertaken by the two PDU directors, and the surrounding environment was relatively stable.

Again, in the early stages the leader had very little involvement in developments outside the unit, although gradually as the PDU itself grew stronger and its work more robust, the role broadened out to include some hospital-wide activity – primarily via involvement in a hospital Clinical Practice Group.

Three years into the PDU, however, this role was radically reviewed. The management structure of the hospital had flattened, causing the senior manager posts formerly associated with the PDU directorships to be further removed from the PDU itself and, as described above, the broader surrounding environment became significantly more changeable. This meant that the leader role needed to increase its political dimensions. As the emphasis of the PDU was shifting towards the need for rigorous, research-based initiatives and the development of research work in priority areas, so the emphasis of the post also needed to shift towards the facilitation of research and practice development, rather than everyday clinical practice on the wards. This was also consistent with the ward sister development programme simultaneously taking place within the hospital, which emphasised the responsibility of the individual ward sisters for leadership of clinical practice within the wards.

In addition the newly defined PDU Leader role bore responsibilities for supporting multidisciplinary development both within the PDU and across the hospital as whole. This change was deliberately implemented to reduce the perception of elitism and isolation associated by some with the PDU, to facilitate dissemination of practice across the hospital and to support the integration of PDU work with other strands of activity – for example clinical audit and business planning.

The right way to define the PDU Leader is one of the areas newly developing units appear to find most difficult. Reflections on this subject have led us to the conclusion that specific clinical leader roles will be as varied as the clinical settings they relate to, and also that just as the philosophy and objectives of the unit need to evolve constantly, so also does the leader role. In broad terms, however, a unit in its early stages of development will be likely to benefit from a more inwardly-focused leader, who has frequent clinical involvement and works directly with staff, motivating and educating. As the unit becomes more mature, the internal activity becomes more self-sustaining, other leaders emerge at the clinical level and a need for a more outward-looking role develops – to disseminate PDU developments, for networking and developing working partnerships, for strategic planning to ensure that benefits of the PDU are maximised across the organisation. Although still important, the balance now needs to shift from sharply clinical, motivational leadership towards a more politically-focused role.

It is important to remember that the PDU is not developing in an entirely neutral environment. A variety of managerial and professional priorities exist, often at odds with one another. It cannot be assumed that a PDU is compatible with all of these agendas. In addition, a PDU is a relatively small and in itself powerless phenomenon. Its own 'power' is derived partly from its track record of achievement, but also (and as importantly) from its capacity to demonstrate real and meaningful connections between different departments' agendas and to address their respective priorities. At the level of the organisation, the PDU does not generate a tidal wave of change. Rather, it is a catalyst for change, creating small reactions here and there, in keeping with its own small scale, which in turn can set off a kind of chain reaction across the organisation as a whole.

Skills of strategic vision, negotiation and political astuteness become vitally important to steer the unit safely into this larger, politically charged arena. If a person could be found who could fulfil all of the potential aspects of the PDU Leader role to an equal degree, that person would be very valuable indeed. In fact, it is likely that leaders with different aptitudes and experience will be needed at different stages of development. No particular type of leader is better than another. The best leader is simply the one who suits best the circumstances and needs of the unit at that time.

Following on from this change in the PDU Leader role, the role of the Research Practitioner was also developed from an existing ill-defined quality role. The purpose of the newly defined role was twofold:

- to help fulfil the goal of the PDU to develop the academic rigour of its work and a portfolio of practice-based research
- to support the leader in facilitating practice development both inside and outside the unit.

This role will be discussed in more detail in Chapter 7. It is worth noting, however, that this implied no shift in terms of resources towards the PDU. With the broadening of the leader role beyond the PDU itself, the unit remained effectively supported by the equivalent of one whole-time person not directly involved in patient care.

In addition to changes in these roles, other developments in the supporting structure and processes of the PDU were instituted, to enable it better to achieve its objectives. These developments are outlined below, but will be discussed in greater detail in the following chapter.

A Steering Group had been established at the outset to provide strategic guidance, influential contacts and high level support. This group was drawn from senior figures both within the host organisation and beyond. In the light of the many changes taking place in the Trust and in the PDU itself, the membership of this group was also reviewed. Members were invited on the basis of the potential relevance of the PDU to their sphere of work and the importance of their support, as well as their high levels of skills, knowledge and experience. Key professional groups relevant to the success of the unit were also included, such as consultants and researchers.

A weekly, multidisciplinary Clinical Forum was established in place of the existing communication meeting, to provide an opportunity for regular clinically-focused discussion and to offset the intensely managerial focus of the organisation as a whole. This forum provided an opportunity for professionals of all disciplines to present work, to discuss ideas, problems or issues, and to communicate with one another. Often ideas arose from these discussions, plans were initiated and multidisciplinary project groups established. Access to these meetings was open to any members of the multidisciplinary team. After its initial establishment, this forum was broadened to involve representation from non-PDU areas. The PDU support systems are illustrated in Figure 3.2.

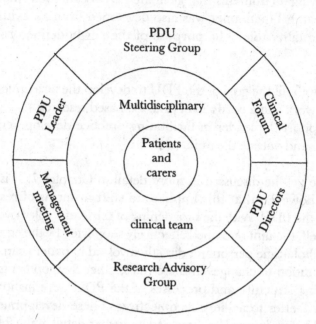

Figure 3.2. PDU support systems.

Links with the Clinical Audit department were fostered via the Clinical Forum, PDU Leader and specific project work. The leader was a member of the hospital Clinical Audit Group and later chaired this group. Similarly, the membership of the Research Advisory Group, established at the outset of the PDU, was also revised and access to its services opened up to staff from any area of the Trust rather than simply from within the PDU itself.

The PDU had always had a separate business plan and action plan to those of the hospital as a whole. However, the unit was managerially part of a larger directorate and therefore a separate business plan was to some extent a notional exercise. Also, this approach tended to emphasise the separateness of the unit, rather than its potential to work for the organisation as a whole and to help it to fulfil its broader objectives. With this in mind, a combined business and action plan was produced, which demonstrated both the distinctive role of the PDU and its integrated contribution to directorate and hospital plans.

Broadly speaking, all of these measures were aimed at integrating the PDU into the organisation as a whole, and at ensuring that the work carried out in the unit could have maximum benefit across the hospital. These developments are discussed in more detail in the next chapter.

Criteria for development units

The final section of this chapter relates to criteria for development units. The King's Fund identified criteria for NDUs and Yorkshire Regional Health Authority similarly specified 15 criteria which NDUs must address in order to achieve accreditation. The latter criteria have subsequently been adapted for use in the accreditation scheme for both NDUs and PDUs facilitated by the Centre for the Development of Nursing Policy and Practice in Leeds (formerly the Institute of Nursing), and are reproduced in Table 3.1 (Institute of Nursing, 1994).

In its early stages, the PDU used these criteria, adapted to a multidisciplinary context, as the basis for discussion of its own philos-

Table 3.1 Criteria for accreditation of development units (Institute of Nursing, 1994)

In order to achieve accreditation, the development unit must:

1   be a defined practice setting
2   have an approach that requires the team to 'opt in'
3   be led by a nurse who acts as consultant and change agent for the nursing team
4   be a place where staff welcome change
5   use its philosphy to determine the conceptual framework for organising nursing practice, incorporating decentralised decision-making and staff empowerment
6   develop staff, utilising a personal development programme
7   have a defined plan of action within a business plan for the NDU which incorporates the process for disseminating evaluated practices
8   operate within baseline resources comparable to clinical care settings in the unit to enable transferability of developments
9   have specific resource requirements related to development
10   evaluate the impact of development in the clinical care setting on the patient, organisation and staff and the environment of care, and inform the Trust Board
11   develop a research-based approach to nursing practice
12   collaborate with higher education to formulate theory and to develop staff
13   collaborate and consult with the multidisciplinary team to achieve patient centred care and to plan developments
14   act as a change agent for nursing practice in the hospital/community, the region, and nationally, publicising its success to promote the value of best practice
15   have a steering group including at least the unit leader, the Trust Chief Nurse, a senior manager and representative of higher education.

ophy and objectives. As described in Chapters 1 and 2, these were helpful in many ways in the early development of the unit. However, even in these early stages of development the PDU had varied certain of these criteria and had pushed others to their limits, making its accreditation a difficult process, with the PDU's interpretation of criteria sometimes at odds with that of accreditors. However, when the time arrived for discussion of a review of the unit's accreditation and a re-evaluation of the unit against these same objectives, it was clear that the unit had developed well beyond such a rigid framework and that the discussion, in fact, threw up more challenges to the accreditation process itself than to the PDU.

What became apparent was that although the same 15 criteria could still broadly be applied to the PDU and be said to inform its philosophy, developments within the unit had rendered the heavy nursing focus of the criteria an even less comfortable fit than originally. Furthermore, within these criteria, which offered a broad definition of a development unit, there could be seen to be considerable scope for variation in specific elements. Many of these possible variations can be seen as differences of balance and emphasis (Table 3.2). These will, of necessity, change over time to reflect changes in internal and external circumstances and influences.

Table 3.2 Elements in balance

Day-to-day care	————————	Change and innovation
Innovation	————————	Consolidation
Practical	————————	Academic
Development	————————	Research
Professional orientation	————————	Service orientation
Pure quality	————————	Value for money
Open agenda	————————	Focused agenda
Independence	————————	Integration

Consideration of some of these elements in more detail will enable us to relate this to the recent and potential development of the unit.

• It is essential to maintain a balance between change and innovation and day-to-day care and quality for the unit's patients. This is, after all, a working unit with real patients. An overemphasis on development at the expense of everyday practice may be perceived as elitist and 'ivory-towered' and may tend to divorce the unit from its patient focus.

- The unit had been a very successful innovator, but not all projects produced lasting changes in everyday practice. There was a need therefore to focus on consolidation of previous ideas as well as development of new ones.
- Work in the unit is essentially practical in nature. However, the matching of this practical focus with increasing academic rigour will only strengthen the quality of the unit's work and increase its value to others outside the unit. With this in mind, measures were taken within the unit to shift the balance slightly towards academic rigour.
- The unit's main focus is on developmental work – developing ideas into practice and ideas from practice. The unit aimed at this stage to maintain its focus on development, but also to move towards more formal research in selected areas by concentrating efforts on specific areas of expertise. One such area was that of stroke rehabilitation.
- The unit has a strong professional orientation. That is, it focuses sharply on clinical and professional issues in patient care. While being keen to maintain this, in order to ensure the unit's relevance to the hospital as a whole, this needed also to be balanced with a broader service focus. This meant, for the PDU, the more explicit inclusion within its remit of non-clinical patient services, and greater consideration of more broadly defined service issues rather than just purely clinical problems.
- Similarly, a focus on pure quality issues needed to be balanced with attention to those of value for money and efficiency. This was essential in order to enable the unit to demonstrate its value to the organisation as a whole where such issues were a priority.
- The unit has an open agenda – all staff can and do shape it. This is an essential part of the PDU ethos. However, in order to develop expertise and the calibre of the unit's work, there was a need to balance this with a more focused approach. For this reason, as well as continuing to vigorously support small scale project work, the unit also began to define specific areas of importance for more detailed attention, many of which would build on previous work. These included stroke rehabilitation, primary nursing and sister development, multidisciplinary documentation, nutrition and ideas related to patient-focused care.
- Finally, there was a need to balance the independence of the unit with its integration into the organisation as a whole. These elements need to be in perfect balance. There is a need to maintain sufficient independence to ensure ideas and innovation are

not stifled. If the agenda of the unit is totally 'given', work on the unit will ultimately lose its relevance to its own patients and the spring of new ideas will dry up.

If, however, work in the unit is totally internally driven and focused, with little thought for the wider world, the unit will be in danger of becoming insular and irrelevant on this broader scale, and therefore be unable to influence or produce benefits outside its own confines.

With the early balance tending towards independence, an important part of the unit's plan for the way forward consisted of looking at ways of shifting this balance slightly the other way.

This process of integration into the broader organisation and approaches to bringing this about will form the subject matter for the next chapter. At this stage in the unit's development, however, it was felt to be essential to its success that it should be an integral part of organisational plans – reflected in business plans and strategy in areas such as research and development, audit, and education and staff development.

Conclusion

This chapter has been about the continued development of the PDU model – a model which continues to develop still.

In the current health service, change has become a way of life and to stand still undoubtedly means to fall behind. What has made the PDU so successful over the years has not been the careful adherence to a list of specific criteria, or the achievement of some ideal state. Rather, it has been its capacity to continuously refresh its underlying principles and to adapt its systems and the focus of its activity, to take into account key developments in the broader organisation and the health service as a whole – without losing sight of these original principles.

A continuous and complex relationship is established between, on the one hand, the unit's philosophy, structure and systems and practical agenda, and on the other, the changes in the broader organisation. Rigid criteria for accreditation in these circumstances only impede growth and stifle innovation.

During the early years of the unit's development, the health service emphasis on multidisciplinary practice increased dramatically, as did the drive towards clinical effectiveness, research-based practice and clinical audit. The ability to address these priorities was essential to the success of the unit. More important still was the ability to respond flexibly to tensions and changes in priority within the hospital as a whole – to ensure that it remained totally relevant to this agenda and played a part in achieving the hospital's objectives. Simple adherence to criteria might be a useful starting point and result in a successful unit in its own terms. However, since development units do not operate in isolation, this is not nearly enough. The performance of development units is, and should be in reality, measured by the yardstick of the broader organisation. Development units clearly cannot afford to become cosy and introspective.

The ultimate conclusion of this chapter, then, could appear to suggest that reading any book or article about development units is futile, and to some extent this may be true. The crucial message to take away is that while there may be a number of broad, common elements of philosophy and approach which tend to underpin all such units, each PDU will, in fact, be unique in any given point in its history. Inevitably then, in a successful unit, responses to this in terms of precise interpretation of principles, infrastructure and methods of support together with the specific focus of its work will also be unique.

As the writing of this book was drawing to a close, the PDU was beginning to undergo a further significant challenge arising from the dramatic changes in the organisation around it after the merger of its hospital with a large, traditional teaching hospital trust. It is unclear at this stage whether even a unit as adaptable as the PDU has proven itself to be, can survive the changes imposed from outside which are materially affecting its operational and professional management, clinical organisation, support structures and systems, and indirectly its culture.

What is clear from this and earlier experiences is that establishment of a PDU at a point in time, although an achievement, is only the beginning. At least as difficult a task is to maintain and develop it further over a period of time. Clarity of vision and a keen political sense are therefore essential in the unit's leaders, together with a constant and energetic attention to the unit's practical and political support.

Chapter 4
Narrowing the gap between practice development and service management

Steve Page

Management and practice development agendas frequently bear little relation to one another, and are often perceived within an organisation as entirely separate issues. This is one of the great frustrations inherent in practice development roles and in any analysis and comparison of such roles between practitioners engaged in them this frustration inevitably emerges. There may often be potential connections between practice development work and the business goals of the organisation, but no mechanism in existence through which these connections can be actively explored. Consequently, there can be difficulties for practice developers in gaining the active interest of managers, and also in ensuring adequate resources for practice development in general as well as for implementation of specific projects. These issues are crucial to ensuring that practice development is both successful in itself and of real value to the organisation as a whole, and therefore should be of concern to both practice developers and managers alike.

Practice developers need the practical support of the organisation to achieve lasting change. They also naturally want to feel that hard work carried out in developing and evaluating practice is going to be seen as relevant by the organisation, and will exert some influence on it. Service managers would perhaps look at the same issue from a different perspective, focused mainly on what resources are going into the activity, what benefits it is going to bring for the organisation and for the quality and cost-effectiveness of its service to patients.

These views will probably not be unfamiliar to those involved in such roles. What is surprising, however, is the difficulty we appear to experience in putting them into practice. Much is made in professional literature of the **research–practice gap**. Perhaps there is also a **practice development–service management gap** which needs to be closed, in order to enable us to maximise our efficiency and effectiveness.

In many organisations the compartmentalisation of practice development and service management is further compounded by the separation of these first two from other discrete entities headed Research and Development (R&D), Quality, Clinical Audit, and so on. Large organisations create artificial divisions between such types of activity, enshrining them in different departments, each with its own hierarchy and distinct set of priorities. Each department develops separately from the others, resulting in rivalries and political game-playing. Great energy is devoted to the creation of precise definitions of each type of activity and projects are perceived to be 'owned' by one department only, with the generation of considerable angst if anyone's toes are felt to have been trodden on. Issues in the care of patients, however, rarely fall neatly into just one of these categories. A truly strategic approach to development must involve a recognition of the major overlaps between these various strands and their integration into one coherent plan, and one of the essential features of good practice development work is that it tends to do just this, softening the boundaries between them.

The emphasis of practice development activity is also firmly on action rather than measurement. This focus on implementation, often within very complex environments, causes practice development to be less tangible than the more easily categorisable activities, such as audit, quality monitoring or research – its results taking more time to achieve and being less easy to present in a 'scientific' format. Some of the great difficulties in practice development, therefore, are to break down the barriers between compartments to facilitate a co-ordinated approach, and also to tap into the resources available to the various 'sexy' and well-funded departments.

This chapter seeks to discuss possible approaches to narrowing the gaps between practice development, service management and other departments, by reference to the work of the PDU. In addition, it will hopefully demonstrate the value to an organisation of the PDU model itself, as a catalyst for bringing these various elements together.

Communication and exchange of ideas

Part of the function of the PDU is to act as a resource for the organisation as a whole. As discussed in the previous chapter, this is of benefit to both the organisation and the unit itself, as development units working solely within their own borders and resources can potentially become stale and insular.

However, attempting to work for the whole organisation can create difficulties for a unit. If the unit functions as the sole 'test-bed' for new ideas or gives the impression of being so, dissemination of its ideas can be perceived to be elitist. It is possible for a unit to exert vast resources and energy in developing and marketing ideas and practice which are not perceived to be meaningful in terms of the organisation's priorities or which cannot immediately be applied.

This development of ideas as project work solely within the confines of the unit and the marketing of ideas as finished products to other areas can also result in the development of feelings of irritation and resentment, as few people enjoy having ideas thrust at them, however good they are. This approach is unlikely to promote the broader 'ownership' of new ideas.

There is also a danger that ideas and practices developed within a unit are directly applicable only to that unit's patients or activity, so that disseminated work appears to be simply of 'academic interest' rather than practical use. If work disseminated by a unit appears consistently to fall into this category, a deep-seated scepticism towards the unit can develop, based on a perception of it as a cosy little place where a protected minority of day-dreamers carry out their pet projects. Clearly, both of these scenarios can be deeply damaging to the unit's potential to bring about change.

With these issues in mind, the PDU sought to broaden the techniques commonly used to disseminate innovations and results of project work. This broader strategy included:

* Establishment of the weekly Clinical Forum to facilitate the exchange of ideas between members of the multidisciplinary team within the PDU. This forum offered opportunity to discuss problems or issues in practice in a non-threatening environment, to air new ideas, to communicate and discuss the implications of ongoing or completed work and to share information between disciplines and individual members of the team. It strongly reinforced the multidisciplinary nature of the PDU and allowed the team to put its stated philosophy into practice, as well as providing a practical vehicle for developmental work.

After its original inception, the forum was expanded further to include representation from other clinical areas around the hospital. This was an important first step for the unit in that this enabled it to discuss PDU ideas and information directly with practitioners from other areas at an early stage, thus helping to ensure the broader relevance of these developments. Equally, it facilitated the inclusion into the unit of ideas and developments from outside its own confines. This helped to ensure that the PDU's agenda remained relevant and refreshed by new ideas. It also sent a powerful message to those outside, that the unit did not perceive itself to be intrinsically better than the rest and that traffic in ideas and innovations was not only one-way.

- In a similar fashion, project groups and pilot exercises established as part of the PDU programme were organised to include representation both from within the PDU and from other areas. Again, this helped to ensure the broader relevance of the developmental work, and also to promote broader 'ownership' of new ideas and practices by avoiding a simplistic 'rational-empirical' change management approach.
- Close collaboration with internal and external educationalists was fostered, to ensure that education and practice development were not seen as mutually exclusive areas. A number of examples demonstrate this principle in action:
  - Involvement of educationalists in development projects in order to enhance the theoretical underpinning of developmental work, and to inform approaches to the introduction of new ideas.
  - Use of the PDU as a site to develop and implement ideas of education professionals.
  - Project work by groups of students linked to PDU agenda.
  - PDU developments supported by education programmes both in-house and delivered by external educationalists.
  - Education programmes routinely informed by PDU developments and project results, for example: multidisciplinary record keeping, discharge workshops, nutrition, special programmes on innovation and change in practice.
- PDU representatives were nominated or selected for inclusion onto a number of hospital and trust-wide groups, including Clinical Audit Groups, Quality Improvement Working Groups and Project Teams, Research and Practice Development forums. In addition, the PDU Leader had a clearly defined role on the directorate management team.

All of the above connections were supported by the design of the PDU Leader role itself. This post, as described in earlier chapters, was developed from the initial Clinical Nurse Specialist-type role, based solely within the unit, to one which now offered support to all disciplines, with an emphasis on change management, facilitation and research skills. In addition, the remit of the postholder was split between the PDU and the rest of the hospital. Half of the role related to support of the PDU itself and was therefore internally focused while the other half was externally focused and related to the development of multidisciplinary practice across the organisation. Clearly, this definition of the role tends strongly to encourage the dissolution of formal boundaries between the unit and other areas.

These measures – open access to PDU discussion forums, cross-membership of project groups and re-definition of the PDU leader role – were decisions which were not as simple as they might appear at first glance. While appearing superficially to contain only positive outcomes for the unit and for the organisation, they did also contain inherent threats to the unit's stability and continued existence. The breakdown of barriers between the PDU and other areas tended to raise difficult and fundamental questions for those working within it:

• What is a PDU?
• How does it differ from other areas if all are involved in the same projects?
• What is the point of a PDU if multidisciplinary practice can be developed in all areas at the same time?

In fact, on closer inspection, it can be seen that such developments arise from the success and maturity of the PDU itself.

In its early stages, a PDU needs to concentrate on developing a culture for innovation and multidisciplinary practice within its own boundaries. However, once the interprofessional boundaries are broken down, the innovative, multidisciplinary culture is well-established within the unit and it is able to feel confident in its own success, then it is ready to begin to break down the barriers between itself and other areas. The strength and energy of the mature PDU team, when linked effectively to the rest of the organisation, is able to drive practice developments on a broader scale. At the same time, the PDU can influence far more widely by fostering a broader sense of ownership and by destroying any sense of elitism or abstraction from reality. Naturally, the PDU team also feeds off ideas from other areas.

As important as the development of specific project work, however, is the capacity for the PDU to inform the broader organisational culture. Much is made of the need to develop positive organisational cultures, focused on teamwork and quality improvement. Bringing individuals from other areas into close contact with a multidisciplinary team in which this culture is already well established will enable them to see and understand the benefits of such an approach. In addition, methods agreed in PDU project teams, driven by the unit's ethos, will be implemented in all areas as part of a specific development project or pilot exercise. This will encourage the development and closer collaboration of new multidisciplinary teams and potentially enable practitioners to experience first hand the benefits of the PDU approach.

In conclusion, then, the PDU must risk loss of its own identity as something separate and therefore risk its own dissolution in order to influence effectively on a broader scale. However, if this risk is successfully managed, the unit's effectiveness in supporting the wider implementation of change in specific clinical practices will be considerably enhanced. Perhaps more importantly still, however, is the capacity for the PDU to influence the culture of the organisation as a whole. The ideal for any organisation must surely be the establishment of a culture in all areas which fosters innovation and quality improvement. The PDU, as an integrated component of an organisational change strategy, offers a practical alternative to the simplistic external consultancy – steering group – educational blitz approach often adopted by organisations as a means of establishing such a culture.

Research and development

A document published by the Yorkshire Regional Health Authority (Yorkshire Health, 1991a) identified three models for supporting R&D in a hospital trust:

- The 'implementation' model, in which the resource is often based in an individual working to a senior nurse or manager, and in which work tends to be progressed through formal channels or groups.
- The NDU model, in which activity is focused within an NDU.
- The 'open access' model, where the research resource is non-hierarchical and open to access by practitioners without prior reference to their superiors, and in which work undertaken reflects the priorities and concerns of practitioners.

In designing the Seacroft Hospital multidisciplinary R&D strategy, a fourth model was created, composed of elements of all these three, with the PDU as a central component. According to this fourth model, the PDU would function both as a testing ground for new ideas for the hospital and as **a** source of R&D support for other areas, the latter principally via the PDU Leader and Research Practitioner roles and from the unit's Research Advisory Group (see Figure 4.1).

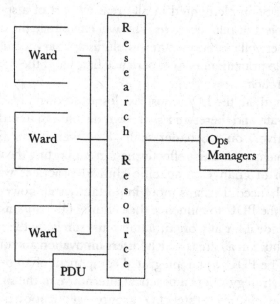

1   Research resource open to approach by all grades and disciplines of staff in the hospital without prior reference to managers or superiors in the first instance.

2   Clear channels of communication between R&D resource, and hospital managers and business planners.

3   R&D activity initiated at both ward, department and managerial level via continuing dialogue.

4   Research resource in the shape of R&D Practitioners and Research Advisory Group with remit to support bottom-up R&D activity, and to facilitate the integration of R&D activity with organisational objectives.

5   PDU functioning as R&D resource and test-bed for new ideas for whole hospital.

6   Links via R&D Practitioners between leadership of PDU and R&D support across site.

Figure 4.1. Model of R&D support. Characteristics of the model. (The model was developed from ideas outlined in Yorkshire Health, 1991b.)

R&D priorities for the hospital would inform the PDU agenda, and vice versa. To ensure that this took place, the PDU team liaised closely with R&D staff working elsewhere in the organisation. In addition, regular input from the broader R&D team to the Research Advisory Group was facilitated

In a King's Fund publication (Vaughan and Edwards, 1995), six models were set out to define the interface between research and practice existing in NDUs. These six models are summarised as follows (although they are acknowledged by the authors not to be mutually exclusive):

* internal evaluation within the NDU team
* researcher as part of the NDU team
* clinical fellows
* unified roles
* external consultants
* external researchers.

Interestingly, only in the conclusion to this text are the following statements made:

> A future model which may be explored is for a clinical unit to act as a central source of expertise for other nurses within the Trust, taking the lead in providing advice and direction to the Trust's overall R&D strategy in relation to nursing issues.

> Much would be gained from such work being undertaken in a multiprofessional context

This is precisely what the PDU has set out to achieve.

All of the NDU models offered by Vaughan and Edwards focus in on the unit itself rather than out towards the organisation as a whole. The development unit is, in other words, the focal point of the model, and the model is designed to effect change within the unit rather than to exert influence beyond its immediate confines. The PDU model, on the other hand, places development clearly in a multidisciplinary context, and the unit as part of a larger system. The internal and external systems of the PDU are intrinsically linked to the function of the broader organisation.

The PDU makes use of all six approaches outlined by Vaughan and Edwards, but also interfaces directly with the organisation as a whole, and with other organisations such as other trusts or universities. If the systems are linked in this way, as one shifts, the others will tend to adjust in order to accommodate. A symbiotic relationship is created, whereby, as the needs of one partner in the relationship change, the other instantly picks these up and reacts to them.

Clinical audit

Within the hospital, clinical audit meetings were held, which had themselves developed from previously existing purely medical audit meetings and from a range of nursing and therapy audit project work. Work carried out within the PDU was presented here, and, similarly, issues were raised which were passed on to the unit's Clinical Forum for further work. This helped to create a direct link between formal clinical audit work and ideas from clinical staff, with three important effects:

- alteration of the perception of clinical audit as something removed from everyday practice
- reinforcement of the multidisciplinary nature of clinical practice
- placement of the emphasis firmly on development (i.e. using audit data to improve practice), rather than on the process of data collection and analysis itself.

An interesting examination is currently taking place of the clinical effectiveness movement with the NHS. Questions are being asked about the apparent failure of the work on systematic reviews, clinical guidelines and protocols to change practice on the ground, in spite of the vast resources ploughed into their development and dissemination.

Those working within the PDU will understand the dynamics underlying this failure. The take-up of clinically effective practices is not dependent solely on their appearing to be good ideas. In addition to this factor are a multitude of issues related to different professional cultures, motivations and priorities, to organisational constraints or inefficiencies and their interactions, and finally to a lack of clarity with regard to boundaries of responsibility at the interfaces between disciplines.

As Harrison (1994) put it in a conference paper, 'to achieve success in change':

> Given that perfect communication and co-ordination within an organisation are unlikely, the number of links in the practitioners' chain of action must be minimal. (A ten-person chain or team, whose individual probabilities of appropriate action are 0.95, has only about a 0.55 probability of perfect implementation).

The vast majority of research into the effectiveness of guidelines is concerned with individual clinical behaviour and cannot confidently be assumed to apply to chains of behaviour – eg, in care packages, inter-agency situations, or even in nursing.

In such team situations, the behaviour of individuals is not independent of the behaviour of colleagues, and others in the relevant social network.

Change of practice may therefore depend on change in the micro-culture of parts of the organisation.

The PDU model helps to address these issues by encouraging the examination of specific areas of clinical care within the multidiscipli-nary context of their actual delivery in practice, rather than as single agency concerns. The PDU philosophy and systems encourage consideration of the real practical implications of material related to clinical effectiveness, be they formal guidelines or protocols or results of in-house clinical audits. The unit's approach and its linkage with clinical audit and R&D departments facilitates the take-up of infor-mation beyond the abstract world of 'good ideas' and into the 'real world' of everyday practices.

As stated in the introduction to this chapter, an imbalance exists between the emphasis and resources afforded the measuring and defining of practice, and those targeted at implementation of this practice. This is probably no accident, in that the former are rela-tively simple and easily demonstrable activities, whereas the latter are inordinately complex and difficult both to define and to evaluate. The PDU offers a practical vehicle for these more complex activities and a means of linking the two broad areas together.

Quality improvement programme

It is not unusual for the consideration of value for money, quality and practice development issues to be led by different managers, and they may each follow entirely different agendas within an organisa-tion. However, within the PDU it is believed that multidisciplinary practice development often has major overlaps with work in the other areas, and can contribute significantly to their aims. For this reason, the unit was seen as an important contributor of ideas and a testing ground for new practices for the organisation's continuous quality improvement programmes.

In the early function of the PDU, project work in the unit was not commonly perceived as having broader cost and quality implica-tions. In fact, the potential for this was present, but either staff were unaware of this, or it had not been effectively demonstrated.

More recent work in the unit includes the following projects (each of which is explained in greater detail in following chapters):

- Continued development of the unit's multidisciplinary records. This included the further development of prompts for interdisciplinary communication within the records themselves; and the removal of layers of overlapping work between disciplines. A further strand of the work entailed the removal of duplication involving two groups of nurses and the medical records department by combining the Reception Unit (similar to Accident and Emergency) card, ward admission notes and medical records admission form into one document. This has implications for efficiency of communication and also for significant reduction of duplicated effort.
- Research into the potential impact of weekend physiotherapy on stroke recovery rates, with obvious implications for length of stay, and therapy resource considerations.
- Pilot implementation of a 'no lifting' policy, designed to reduce the incidence of back injury among nurses and other professionals.

Each of these pieces of work, while clinically led, can of course readily be seen to have quality and value for money implications. These implications are now explicitly stated at the outset of any PDU project work and also inform its evaluation. In this way, the work of the PDU can clearly be seen to be related to organisational priorities of efficiency, cost-effectiveness and value for money. This is, of course, essential in an NHS environment of increasing resource constraint, where a failure to address these priorities results in an 'ivory tower' image and rapid sidelining of a unit's activity.

In addition, a hospital-wide project, officially under a Continuous Quality Improvement banner, was led by the PDU Leader and although involving eight disciplines and departments, both clinical and non-clinical, was clearly seen to be driven by the PDU ethos and energy. This project work related to the multifaceted subject of dealing with a patient's death addressed clinical issues related to the patient after death (last offices, transport, storage), the needs of the family (viewing, comfort, information and advice) and the administrative needs of the organisation. In doing so, it demonstrated both the complex connections and interdependencies between the multidisciplinary clinical and non-clinical elements of the hospital services, and the capacity of the PDU to act as a catalyst to bring these two together and to address issues of both quality and efficiency.

Business planning

Commonly, the business planning process is viewed and enacted as something entirely separate from practice development. However, clinical practice developments must be resourced if they are to be successful; and usually new clinical developments will have broader financial or service delivery implications. In the PDU it has been found that failure to make this practical link between the two areas can have damaging results. If the clinical imperative is sufficiently powerful (often this relates to power of the individual practitioner or professional group rather than to the persuasiveness of the practice itself) then the new practice is implemented in spite of a lack of resources to support it. In effect, resources are usually diverted from another area. If, however, the clinical imperative is not sufficiently powerful and the risks to the organisation in not implementing the change do not appear great, then the practice may not be fully implemented, with a negative impact on quality of care and morale of the staff involved in developing and piloting the new practice.

An example of this from within the unit was the development of a self-medication scheme for older patients. The purpose of this scheme was to enable patients to develop their understanding of their medication and the skills to administer this safely, prior to discharge. The study was one of the earliest instances of multidisciplinary collaboration within the unit and between the PDU and the local university. It also received regional funding and was published via a number of journal articles and conference papers.

The study provided evidence to demonstrate a greater understanding of and 'compliance' with their drug prescriptions, after discharge, of patients in the experimental self-medication group as compared with those in the control group.

However, the full implementation of this scheme after the cessation of the pump-priming project money, was dependent on the funding of a part-time pharmacy technician and a few hours of pharmacist time per week. Unfortunately, this resource implication had not been identified at the outset, and subsequently this led to the abandonment of the new practice at the close of the research study and to a protracted battle for additional funds. The impact of this on the morale of the unit's team cannot be overestimated.

The current approach of the unit in seeking to integrate its programme of developments with business plans of the hospital as a whole, is at least in part aimed at preventing a recurrence of this situation.

The accreditation body to which the PDU was initially affiliated required the unit to formulate a business plan of its own, which was separate from that of the larger organisation. While probably designed primarily to protect development units, this also has two less desirable effects. First, the business plan created can tend to be somewhat artificial, as multidisciplinary development units tend to be entities which cut across managerial and budgetary boundaries and whose existence is based more on shared philosophy and collaborative working than on formal structures. Second, this emphasises the position of the unit as external to the organisation as a whole. In order to bring business planning and practice development activity closer together, the unit elected to move on from this approach and, while retaining the distinct 'flavour' of the PDU, has integrated its planning into that of the clinical directorate and hospital as a whole. The subsequent business plans have stated explicitly how the PDU is seen to fit into the whole, and the unit's action plan forms part of the broader programme, endorsed and actively supported by managers. This approach helps to maintain the vibrancy of the business plan and ensures its relevance to patient need, while also providing ideas to stimulate new developmental work with the PDU.

Conclusion

Development units are celebrated and well-supported by those involved in their activities and have been publicised widely. Elitism has, of course, always been seen as a danger for such units which deliberately set out to be innovative. However, a more real and pressing danger for such units is that of irrelevance.

A fundamental justification for development units is that they should function as a resource for the broader organisation. On a simple level, this consists of sharing ideas, dissemination of results and 'selling' of improved practices to other areas. The PDU has sought to develop beyond this simplistic approach. There is great potential within the multidisciplinary working of the unit for exploring broader service issues and interfaces between disciplines. The aim has been to draw on this potential to enable the unit to fulfil more effectively its organisational resource role. The PDU's approaches to project work draw on accepted change theory to enhance the relevance of its work to other areas, and to increase the likelihood of its uptake. By facilitating (through the development of its systems, roles and methods of work) close communication and exchange of ideas between the unit and other areas, the PDU has integrated itself more effectively into wider planning and development, and has therefore helped to increase its relevance to broader organisational goals.

Most areas could potentially work in the PDU style (although naturally each would need to adapt the general principles to suit its own specific needs). One of the reasons for initiating the development unit model, however, is to enable an organisation to concentrate its resources in one area to start with, rather than dissipating them across a vast area. The outward-looking approach of the unit to management and leadership described above offers a mechanism of moving beyond this initial concentration to the support of lasting change in the wider organisation, as much by helping to spread the underlying learning culture as through resulting project work.

It is likely that a newly created unit needs to concentrate its resources on inward development to start with, until it has achieved a critical mass of committed practitioners, a stable culture and system and can point to a number of practical successes. Organisations need to be patient and supportive of a unit through this stage, before significant broader benefits can be achieved. It is essential to the continued development of the unit, however, that once this stage is reached it does not become fixed. Units which have become fixed in the inward-focused mode after their initial stage of implementation tend not to be able to demonstrate fulfilment of their broader organisation role, and have consequently fallen by the wayside or been more readily abandoned by their host hospitals.

PDUs are a relatively new phenomenon and not everyone is clear about the differences between the PDU and NDU approaches. However, one of the most important manifestations of this difference is in the greater potential of PDUs to contribute to and draw together different agendas across the organisation. (The differences between PDU and NDU models are discussed more fully in the next chapter.)

In conclusion, current issues in the health service include an all-pervading concern with cost effectiveness and value for money; an increasing concern with clinical effectiveness and the riddle of how to achieve it in practice (currently attempted largely in vain via university and Trust R&D and Clinical Audit departments); and a growing interest in new approaches to contracting underpinned by multidisciplinary pathways of care spanning hospital and community. The PDU model is designed to support all of these developments and to act as a catalyst to link together the work on these various strands towards one common goal – improvement in patient care.

Ultimately, however, a PDU or any other unit can only achieve this catalytic potential in a large NHS trust if the senior managers of the organisation have the vision to appreciate this and offer their support to overcome the many powerful, vested interests inherent in the organisation's departments and professional groups – many of which are at odds with the very concept of integration discussed in this chapter.

In the hospital environment in which the PDU became established and functioned for its first five years, managers of the organisation as a whole were receptive to such ideas and played an active role in promoting collaboration between different departments and professions. This was important in helping to create the kind of atmosphere in which the PDU could function at its best. It remains to be seen whether the unit will be able to continue this role as catalyst within a larger and significantly more traditionally oriented NHS trust organisation, where demarcation and compartmentalisation of spheres of responsibility and activity, and organisation within strictly professional hierarchies, are the norm.

Chapter 5
PDUs and NDUs:
a comparison

David Allsopp

This chapter describes the history and origins of nursing development ment units (NDUs), especially those at Tameside, Burford and Oxford. The aims and key principles of NDUs are presented and discussed in comparison with the Seacroft Practice Development Unit (PDU). Earlier chapters described how the Seacroft PDU evolved with an emphasis on multidisciplinary working, with development driven by the needs of patients. This approach differs markedly from that taken by nursing development units, although there are some common features, especially regarding the promotion of quality care, empowerment of staff and patients and the need to be innovative in developing practice.

After an examination of the advantages and disadvantages of the PDU and NDU approaches in relation to effective multidisciplinary team working, organisational influence and developing nursing, the chapter discusses the benefits of PDUs for the wider organisation, such as a raised profile for the trust, a source of innovation, a test-bed for new approaches and a research profile. The chapter concludes with reference to the trend for NDUs to begin calling themselves PDUs.

The history and origins of NDUs

One of the first NDUs established in the UK began life at Burford near Oxford following the appointment of Dr Sue Pembrey as a clinical practice development nurse in the Oxford Health Authority and

Alan Pearson as nursing officer at Burford in 1981 (Pearson, 1983). There were often particular local circumstances which drove the establishment of NDUs, as there were later at Seacroft. In the case of Burford, there was a need to find ways of developing a small community hospital under threat of closure, to make it more economical and to update its ethos. The chief nurse recognised that nursing had a valuable contribution to make to the sort of changes which were necessary at Burford and was keen to take a chance that Alan Pearson could swing things round.

The approach taken at Burford was influenced by the work of Lydia Hall at the Loeb Centre in New York, and centres at Rush University and Rochester University, USA. The Loeb Centre for Nursing, set up as a center of excellence as early as 1963, used nursing as the main therapy, working with medicine and other disciplines rather than being subservient to them. The importance of a healing role for nursing was stressed. 'Centres of excellence' at Rush and Rochester Universities had developed new extended nursing roles and there was an emphasis on the integration of nursing practice, education and research.

Pearson describes the aim of the 'clinical nursing unit' as promoting

> high quality nursing and, in doing so, the development of clinical nursing as a discipline through its practice, education and research. Its activities focus on nursing as a therapeutic agent. . . . The practice of nursing in the clinical nursing unit must be based on the healing potentials embodied in the acts of nursing' (Pearson, 1983).

Stephen Wright and colleagues also established a highly influential NDU in 1987 at Tameside Hospital on the edge of Manchester. Purdy *et al.* (1988) describe the creation of the NDU at Tameside as born out of the desire to change their traditional approach to elderly care, whose low status was seen as inhibiting recruitment and retention of staff. There were no high profile medical specialties or techniques, but staff were keen to improve nursing and saw the provision of management which encouraged and supported by providing opportunities for staff development as crucial to success. Drawing on the work of Orton (1981) on ward learning climate, the team at Tameside saw how working climate was determined by the manager.

> Staff need to feel encouraged, with opportunities to continue their learning. In an atmosphere where the manager is more inclined to say yes than no, to be libertarian rather than controlling, to be democratic rather than autocratic, staff can feel secure, nourished and valued (p. 34).

Purdy continues:

> The supportive climate of our organisation can foster innovation
> which, in turn, brings new stimulus and challenge to nurses. Nurses feel
> rewarded when they feel they are succeeding; that standards of patient
> care are being achieved; that patient satisfaction is high; and that care is
> being improved.

The Tameside team identified several principles necessary for
success. These included:

- access to opportunities for personal development through a
  rolling programme organised with the support of the continuing
  education department
- sticking to plans laid
- funding
- peer support through groupings of various sorts
- evaluation to assess progress and provide feedback.

The benefits of this approach were illustrated by the fact that Tameside NDU had a waiting list for nurses by 1989.

The NDU on Beeson ward at Oxford's Radcliffe Infirmary, led
by Dr Sue Pembrey (a nurse), was closed down in March 1989 after
three and a half years, having failed to convince managers of the
value of the approach. This was despite evidence of high standards
of care, innovative work and research and strong patient support
(Salvage, 1992). This NDU was a unit of 16 'nursing beds', to which
patients were admitted once their need for medical intervention had
passed. Admission and discharge were nursing decisions.

At the same time as the Oxford NDU closure, the King's Fund
Centre was offering pump priming grants totalling £531 500 to set
up and support NDUs for three years, and units at Brighton,
Camberwell, Southport and West Dorset were successful in their
bids of up to £90 000 each. By 1992, the Department of Health was
also funding 28 NDUs around the country (Christian and Redfern,
1996).

Often the interest in setting up NDUs came from nurses themselves. It was very much a 'bottom up' initiative of the sort increasingly seen as a desirable part of an enabling, devolutionary
management style. The same was true for the Seacroft PDU in that
the drive came from middle manager level, with support from the
unit general manager, the clinical director who had a strong interest
in management, and from clinical staff. The unit general manager at

the time of the move from St George's was quite happy to allow managers to manage as they saw fit, and if this meant starting a PDU that was fine as long as managerial objectives were achieved.

What exactly is an NDU?

Nursing development units aim to become

> centres of nursing excellence in their hospital, neighbourhood or health authority. They launch and evaluate experiments in good practice, supported by sound education, management and research. Close relationships with other health staff are also fostered. (Salvage and Black)

They are based on the idea that the culture of practice is underpinned by nursing values and beliefs. One of these is a reluctance to see a clear distinction between 'care' and 'cure':

> high quality nursing not only makes patients more comfortable, mentally and physically, but also plays an active role in restoring them to health or enabling them to achieve their maximum potential.

In other words, NDUs were seeking to realise the therapeutic potential of nursing as something which was a proactive force for health, not just a follower of others' prescriptions: 'One advantage of an NDU is that it raises the profile of nursing within a health authority, and thereby helps to explain to the public, managers and doctors how the nursing role is changing from passive caring to active healing' (King's Fund Centre, 1993).

The role of NDUs in the development of nursing as a profession

The desire of nursing to become a 'true' profession is one which has been growing over the last few decades, as nurses have sought to break out from medical dominance and to assert themselves as independent practitioners. This aspiration is based on a belief that nurses can make a unique contribution to improving health which does not rely on them following others' treatment prescriptions. 'Nurses are recognising that they too are healers and facilitators who allow the patients to heal themselves' (McMahon, 1991). If nursing can make a unique contribution to improving health, the argument goes, then it is ripe for becoming a proper profession. The changes in nurse education since the 1970s have seen a move into higher education, with a development also of much interest in nursing research. If there is something special about what nurses do, then it should be researched so as to add to the body of knowledge required of a profession. One NDU stated clearly that their mission was 'to raise the profile of nursing as a profession' (Bamford *et al.*, 1990).

Cole and Vaughan (1994), in a review of successful applicants for NDU status described a vision common to them all that an NDU was 'a nursing-led initiative to demonstrate what nursing can offer' (Director of Nursing, Brighton). Success would enhance nursing's credibility. The Southport mission statement said 'in fulfilling this aim [of improving patient care], it is hoped that the status of nursing will be raised, so it can be identified as a legitimate and valued specialty.'

Similarly, Turner-Shaw and Bosanquet (1993) in their report on two and a half years progress at the four King's Fund NDUs commented that

'I . . . hope that the NDU will really show the potential of nursing and the contribution of nursing in the care of elderly people requiring health care.

The NDU and particularly the attainment of King's Fund Centre support was 'seen as a means of giving nurses new thrust' (Nurse Manager), particularly in medically dominated environments with little promotion of nursing as a discipline, and in those areas perceived as having low status because of the high percentage of elderly patients'.

The report recommended that NDUs

'should be considered by any health care organisation seeking to provide effective, high quality care to patients and clients. Such units provide a way of developing nurses and their practice within finite resources' (p. 1).

Twelve other recommendations were made, concerned mainly with how best to make NDUs a success. No recommendation was made about the need to consider multidisciplinary involvement in an NDU, despite the finding that other professionals, especially doctors, had felt poorly informed about NDUs and their purpose. Nurses had appreciated 'the need to inform and involve other disciplines' (p. 17) but had found 'little opportunity to meet regularly with other disciplines, particularly doctors, to discuss non-clinical aspects of team work.'

Threats to interprofessional cooperation

One of the implications of a focus on the development of nursing is the sense of threat this could create amongst other professions. Physiotherapists, occupational therapists and other colleagues are relatively few in number and have their own concerns about the status of their professions. For nurses to declare a ward as a nursing-led unit with the aim of developing nursing could be damaging to professional relationships and effective team working. In a letter to *Nursing*

Times, Wright (1997) recognises that interprofessional relationships must be handled sensitively, but argues that nurses should not hold back from seeking NDU status even if this 'rocks the boat' and upsets other disciplines. 'If others have a problem when nursing clarifies and asserts itself, then that is just the point – it is their problem.' Such an attitude seems to miss the point. How can it be in the best interests of patients if interprofessional relationships are damaged? Surely nurses need to learn to develop their practice, and by all means celebrate their achievements, within the context of the team of which they are a part.

Indeed, perhaps the fact that nurses are prepared to engage in discussions about practice development with other professions without feeling the need for some form of more segregated development indicated something else. As Ford and Walsh (1994) said:

> Nurses might feel worried about the loss of nursing as a distinct entity within this approach. The anti-nursing, anti-professional bias of many senior managers in the NHS today makes this totally reasonable. One approach might be initially to carry out research which does focus in a narrow sense on the value of nursing before moving on to a more integrated approach. Perhaps it will be a sign of real nursing maturity and empowerment when we feel confident in taking our place within such a multidisciplinary team and concentrate on measuring the improvement in the quality of the patient's life which results from a team approach to care.

Nursing is operating in a complex, multidisciplinary, multiagency health care system. In such a context, there are few issues which could be described as purely nursing. For many medical patients in hospital the concern is about how to successfully rehabilitate for return home or to some other care setting. This is very much a multidisciplinary team affair, with few aspects over which nurses have sole control.

- Mobilising is a shared responsibility between nurses and physiotherapists.
- Nurses and occupational therapists share involvement in washing and dressing practice.
- Nurses, doctors, occupational therapists and social workers combine their efforts in discussing plans for discharge with families.

If a problem arises it is hard to see how it can be tackled if not by the relevant members of the multidisciplinary team getting together to seek solutions. What about taking things even further and involving patients and their relatives in defining the problems and suggesting

solutions? In such a multidisciplinary setting there seemed at
Seacroft to be no other way to proceed. Changes in practice had to
be driven by the needs of patients. What was sought was an
approach which recognised the value of all members of the team
(including the patient), which was interested in the quality of ideas
not who suggested them, and which sought to provide the sort of
working culture and environment which released people's energy
and encouraged collaboration.

For reasons such as these, some units have called themselves
PDUs not NDUs, although there has still been a concern with the
role of nursing. A statement in 1991 on PDUs says

> In multidisciplinary settings it may be sensible to call such a unit a Prac-
> tice Development Unit – recognising that nurses would still take the
> lead (Yorkshire Health, 1991b).

Although the emphasis in the Seacroft PDU was different to the NDU
approach, there is much they have in common. There is a shared
belief that the philosophy of care should be developed collectively and
should be underpinned by a shared vision of high quality practice.
There is a commitment to equity and equality, and wanting to increase
the involvement of patients and their relatives in decision making
regarding care and treatment. Seacroft staff saw the inevitability of
change and wanted a 'proactive, dynamic, challenging and planned
approach to the management of change'. There is also a desire for
'individual practitioner autonomy', with opportunities for empowerment and development. The development of research-based practice
is a key feature for the PDU as well, although Seacroft wanted to take
things further by conducting research itself whenever possible. Evaluation of innovation is important, particularly in testing the effectiveness
and efficiency of care and treatment, and research is an important
strand of evaluation. Perhaps above all there is a need to disseminate
the results of work. The success of the model in influencing practice
development in the organisation as a whole depended on this. The
PDU was not an end in itself. Without effective dissemination the work
was pointless. The PDU was a 'laboratory for change', and once the
value of some change to practice had been demonstrated, the next
step was to influence change in other parts of the hospital and beyond.

By virtue of their numbers nurses would have a lot of influence in
shaping the PDU approach, but there were other influences too,
including organisational development theory contributed by
managers, and the aspirations and approaches to work of other
professional groups.

Similarities and differences between NDUs and PDUs

There are more ways in which NDUs are similar to PDUs than different. The key principles of NDUs (King's Fund Centre, 1995) are set out in Table 5.1, in comparison with statements from the philosophy and aims of the Seacroft PDU.

Table 5.1 NDU principles and PDU philosophy and aims

NDU principles	PDU philosophy and aims
An approach that increases the involvement of patients/clients in decision making regarding their own care	We believe that patients have the right to be involved in decisions about their care and that we should work towards empowering them to participate fully
Empowerment and development of individual nurses	Aims to promote accountability and autonomy of individual professions in a multidisciplinary framework
A high level of individual practitioner autonomy	Aims to continue to develop a management style which is supportive and which promotes the involvement of staff at appropriate levels of decision making
Acceptance by staff of change as a way of life, and of a proactive, dynamic, challenging and planned approach to the management of change	The PDU is a centre for innovative, creative practice where change for the better is accepted as an essential feature of development
	We wish to promote a questioning attitude to all aspects of practice and recognise that there is a need to accept well-considered risk taking as part of development
	Aims to encourage new approaches to patient treatment, care and therapy
A philosophy of care which is developed collectively and is underpinned by a shared vision of high quality nursing practice, and espouses the values of equity and equality in care	We value the contribution of all members of the multidisciplinary team in promoting high quality care and practice development
	Aims to provide high quality, effective care for all patients
Development of research-based practice	We encourage research-based practice and support its development through education and clinically based research projects
	Aims to support research within the PDU
Sharing of new ways of practice	We recognise that the PDU has a wider responsibility to encourage and support development in the unit as a whole
	Aims to promote strong links with educational institutions
Evaluation of effectiveness and efficiency of nursing care	Aims to agree appropriate methods of evaluating change
	We believe that success depends on positive results which benefit patients

Empowerment of patients

Both NDUs and PDUs share a strong commitment to the involvement of patients in the decision-making process. For the PDU this was addressed partly through the encouragement of patients to read and comment on multidisciplinary care plans, through research which sought their views about the service, and their involvement in discussions about their care after discharge. This is discussed further in Chapter 9.

Empowerment of staff

The empowerment and development of individual nurses is a key issue for NDUs. Empowerment in the PDU means encouraging staff to take responsibility for their actions and decisions as far as is reasonably possible. People closest to the problem often have an idea about how best to solve it. Primary nursing is one way in which nurses are empowered to make decisions and is as much a part of the PDU approach as it is in NDUs. For the PDU the concern was with the promotion of accountability and autonomy of all members of the team. There was also a recognition that good ideas could come from any source at any level, so that if a physiotherapy assistant had a suggestion it should be judged on its merit, not according to who put it forward. Leadership of projects would also depend, not on being a member of a particular profession, but on who had the right skills and knowledge. This requires a management style which supports the devolution of decision making and responsibility, something common to NDUs and the PDU, but operationalised differently in each.

The issue of practitioner autonomy was also a shared concern. For NDUs the focus was on nursing autonomy, a very real issue in terms of the development of nursing as a profession. This is one of the key defining features of independent nursing practice which almost alone prevents nursing from claiming true professional status.

In the PDU, staff development is seen as important, but it is equally so for therapy professions, who often have few or no resources to support staff development. The PDU has been able to find ways of supporting professional development amongst therapy colleagues, such as by involving them in research and collaborative audit activity. The PDU is also supported by a continuing education department which provides opportunities for training and development for staff from all professional and other backgrounds.

The development of effective team functioning is also relevant to both approaches. What differs perhaps is the definition of who is in 'the team'. In practice, staff are members of several different teams all at once, some clearly defined and others less so. The PDU seeks to encourage everyone involved in patient care directly or indirectly to think of themselves as team members. This can be quite difficult, as accountability is not always to the same person. What remains important, however, is that all have the patient as the common focus, that the team has clearly defined aims and works together towards achieving them. This is discussed further in Chapter 8.

The pressures of change

The need to see change as a permanent feature is something shared closely by NDUs and the PDU, as was the belief in being proactive, dynamic, challenging, and having a planned approach to change. Development could not happen without change taking place. It was important to avoid change for its own sake, placing an emphasis on 'change for the better'. An important feature of identifying the need for change was to encourage a questioning attitude to practice and to allow well-considered risk taking as part of development activity. In other words, if someone had an idea for a change to clinical practice, the first step was to establish baseline measures of what was happening. Introducing the change would involve a certain risk that the idea would not work. It is essential that risks be anticipated as far as possible and minimised or removed all together.

Commitment to quality

NDUs and the PDU are strongly committed to providing quality care. The difference lies in the means. For NDUs the focus of attention is upon ensuring high quality nursing care. The PDU approach is to see this as important too, but as part of a wider picture which sees the nursing contribution as part of a team effort. Nursing does not function in isolation from other professions, but must coordinate its activities with those of others to ensure effective and efficient team working. Nursing will certainly have a vital role in terms of coordination and communication, and is also unique in being the only professional grouping which has 24 hour contact with patients. Consequently, the quality of nursing is a fundamentally important part of quality patient care.

   The PDU ethos certainly supported the notion of developing a philosophy of care collectively. Where it differs is in the nature and extent of collective involvement. At Seacroft right from the start it was a multidisciplinary debate. All the discussions and time-out sessions and standard-setting activity focused on developing a multidisciplinary philosophy of quality care. This did not mean that individual professions could not also aspire and work towards developing their own practice; this happened too. In addition, by addressing issues of multidisciplinary team effectiveness, the PDU was tackling concerns about equity of access which were also of concern to NDUs. For the PDU there was much more concern about how different professions related to each other and worked together, and how responsibilities overlapped; about how communication should work, about team goals and strategies for achieving them.

Development of research-based practice

The recognition of the need for research-based practice has been something which has driven both NDU and PDU activity. Work on promoting an appreciation of the value of research is now bearing fruit as increasing attention is being given to concerns about clinical effectiveness. This is discussed further in Chapter 12. For the moment, it is sufficient to say that the emphasis in NDUs is very much about nursing research. It is by conducting research into the value of nursing that NDUs aim to assist the process of professionalisation of nursing. For this to be achieved a knowledge base for nursing derived through research is essential. The PDU does not preclude nursing research from taking place; on the contrary, it is welcomed if nurses want to do research into nursing. The difference lies in the argument that nursing has to sort out where it fits with everything else. It cannot isolate itself from the rest of the world for several years while it sorts itself out. The argument that nurses need to work alone to build their confidence before entering the fray has some merit, but it was felt in the PDU that it was better to get 'stuck in' right from the start. The PDU sought a more collaborative approach, conducting research on issues of relevance to the multidisciplinary team. It was interesting to see how more recently much emphasis has been given to research which is multidisciplinary, multiagency or multisite. This is driven by the need for seekers of research funds, particularly at universities, to meet such criteria to be successful in their bids. Ways in which the PDU supported research are discussed in Chapter 7.

Dissemination of good practice

Dissemination of good practice is a major concern of both NDUs and PDUs. The PDU model takes dissemination very seriously, seeing it as more than just the spreading of information about achievements, important though this is. It is also about encouraging the dissemination of the cultural and organisational features which support practice development. The idea of having a special unit or ward in which ideas are developed and then spread through the rest of the organisation will only work if there is real commitment from the organisation to that model of working.

The NDU and PDU approach is to place a strong emphasis on staff involvement, training and development, with support concentrated at ward level. Individuals are encouraged to make decisions for themselves when faced with particular problems, without having to refer to higher authority. This is one of the main reasons for employing professionals in the first place, and incidentally, why the dilution of skill mixes makes it harder to maintain quality care.

The usual approaches to dissemination of good practice include seminars, internal newsletters, publication in journals, conferences and study days, visits from interested enquirers etc. The PDU has used all of these and has been quite successful because of this in raising the name of Seacroft around the region and beyond. It is not clear to what extent such publicity resulted in the wider adoption of innovation. (See Chapter 11 for a further discussion of this point.)

Within one's own trust, it is always more difficult to sell ideas. This is where the internal politics can make life a little more complicated. Approaches which take a centralist, bureaucratic view of life by having non-clinically based departments issuing 'top down' policies will struggle to succeed, especially in large hospitals. Of course there is a need to ensure that certain standards are maintained across the trust on some issues. On others, standards will be relevant only to specific clinical areas. Innovations developed in a unit such as a PDU may be irrelevant to other parts of the hospital. What is relevant is the way in which problems are tackled effectively. The PDU is basically a way of promoting a team approach to problem solving.

As well as aiming to encourage the spread of innovation to other clinical areas, the PDU also sees it as important to try and influence educators in local universities and colleges. PDU staff have cultivated links with lecturers in higher education to promote a two-way cross-fertilisation of ideas. Nursing students have worked in the PDU as 'syndicate students' to develop and implement local clinical guidelines with PDU staff, who in turn have contributed to teaching in the university.

Evaluation

For NDUs the focus of evaluation is on the effectiveness and efficiency of nursing care. Whilst the PDU shares this aim, a broader perspective is also important. Evaluation of change has always been a key element of PDU activity in the sense that it is seen as essential to be able to demonstrate the value of work done in the unit. Evaluation has therefore usually related to assessing the extent to which projects achieve their stated objectives. A variety of methods are used as part of the audit process, and the PDU is also keen on using research as a means of evaluation whenever possible, although this requires greater resources. Increasingly, the PDU is addressing the need to evaluate effectiveness and efficiency issues. This is driven in part by the desire to take on board the messages about the need for clinical effectiveness, and also by the need to demonstrate to managers that the PDU is efficient in its use of resources and provides value for money. The use of cost–benefit analyses, whilst desirable, is a highly complex task which requires considerable knowledge and skill. It is perhaps easier to measure the costs of an innovation and somewhat more difficult to measure the benefits, which are often qualitative in nature. The PDU has begun some research into the views of newly diagnosed diabetics to find out what their views of the service are. The intention is to use the results of this evaluation to inform service provision. This is described in more detail in Chapter 12.

Clinical leadership

It is a requirement of NDUs that the unit is led by a nurse. Who else could lead on the development of nursing? In the Seacroft PDU all three (plus one acting) clinical leaders have been nurses, although there has never been a requirement that a nurse was appointed. They were known as PDU leaders, not nurses. Anyone with the right range of skills could have been appointed. What mattered more was a commitment to multidisciplinary practice development. In practice it is difficult for members of therapy professions to apply for such a post, as it does not fit easily into therapy career ladders. There is no clear or easy route for therapists after they move on from such a post.

The concern that nurses should lead everything seems to miss the point that what is most important is that leadership should surely come from the most appropriate source. It depends on the issue. It may be politically expedient that a project is led by a medical consultant, whereas for other things leadership may best come from physiotherapists, dietitians or nurses. If nurses try to lead everything they may find themselves meeting more resistance to change.

The clinical setting and its workforce

NDUs have almost all been based on one ward or department with a nursing team which works exclusively on that ward. Although there may be some lending of staff to other wards to cover staffing problems, and the use of agency or bank nurses, the nursing team is 'static'. On a PDU, more than one ward may be included (as is the case at Seacroft). This is because of the work patterns of the different therapists involved in patient care. Physiotherapists, occupational therapists and others see patients on more than one ward. Their more mobile work patterns mean that they are part of more than one team. There is then a need to see the PDU as a larger setting than just one ward to allow for this fact. Of course this makes everything more complicated, but it was felt to be the appropriate way forward. The other issue then becomes whether practice development can be supported across several different wards at once. This was in fact one of the concerns the King's Fund Centre had when considering the PDU's early bid for funds. The proposal was to include four 24 bed wards in the PDU, supported by one clinical leader and the quality assurance nurse for the hospital.

Vision and philosophy

Since the focus in NDUs is on nursing, all of the NDU team are from the same profession, which is at a particular stage of its development. On a PDU a range of professions with different histories, at different stages of development and with differing philosophies are part of the team.

PDUs and NDUs: advantages and disadvantages

The perceived advantages and disadvantages of the two approaches will depend on perspective, of course. Those wishing to see nursing taking a leading role, with specific emphasis on developing new knowledge about nursing to support the development of nursing as a profession, will be more likely to support an NDU approach. The NDU provides a relatively safe haven where nurses can develop their knowledge, skills and confidence before engaging in 'real world' debates. This can be a real advantage, as the effect of exposing young, enthusiastic, politically naive nurses to the rigours of organisational politics can be very damaging. One can only admire those nurses who have developed their management and leadership skills to get the best out of others and who are able to articulate clearly the value of the contribution of nursing to patient care. The contribution of NDUs to advancing the knowledge base of nursing and the testing of new approaches has been outstanding. Nurses are quite right to be proud of their achievements. In addition, NDUs have done much to raise the status of elderly care, as at Tameside (Black, 1993), although there is no reason why this could not also happen in a PDU.

The sorts of developments seen in NDUs, such as in the use of bedside handovers, pain management, use of a carers' panel and a patients' forum, nutritional awareness and wound care, have been well documented (Black, 1992). With the exception of wound care all of these have also been tackled in the Seacroft PDU. All are issues which have multidisciplinary relevance except bedside handovers. The NDU approach may limit the extent to which nursing can develop since it creates an apparently artificial situation of pretending that other professions are not there, or if they are it is not on an equal footing.

The advantages of the PDU approach are that developments in practice are driven by the needs of patients not professional aspirations. This is not to say that NDUs are not concerned with improving patient care, of course they are; but as Cole and Vaughan said of one NDU 'it has been found to be more effective to concentrate negotiation around patient need rather than nursing development, as this is less threatening and indeed is the fundamental reason behind the work' (Cole and Vaughan, 1994).

The PDU makes a point of encouraging multidisciplinary team work. Staff from different professions and disciplines are deliberately brought together to tackle problems and see each other as equal members of a team. Such joint working recognises the contribution of all disciplines and all levels of staff to developing new ideas and encourages a non-hierarchical relationship between professions. The PDU provides opportunities for multidisciplinary collaboration on audit and research and promotes understanding of different roles through the discussion of the boundaries between professions. Opportunities to influence managerial agendas may be increased by having a strong multidisciplinary team (which includes managers).

One disadvantage of the PDU approach is that the scale of involvement of different disciplines makes for greater complexity. However, few problems are simple anyway, and the PDU makes an honest attempt to recognise this by involving all relevant staff or their representatives. Another problem is that PDU staff may be responsible to a range of different managers or even be attached to different directorates – not necessarily on the same hospital site – making cooperation potentially difficult. Some professionals may see it as problematic if a PDU is led by someone with a nursing background. This was not the case at Seacroft, where all PDU leaders have been nurses, although two could have come from any background. Finally, involving therapists in projects can place excessive demands on them as they are relatively few in number compared with nurses.

PDUs – organisational benefits

The benefits for a trust having a development unit, whether it be NDU or PDU, can be considerable, although they are not always fully appreciated. The experience of Oxford NDU is a lesson in how even high profile units are not immune from closure, having failed to convince managers of their value.

Perhaps the most notable benefit for the wider organisation is that the PDU provides a model of how health services can begin to address issues of effectiveness of care and treatment. These are not just concerns about choosing the right drug or the most appropriate surgical intervention, but are about how the service as a whole selects and delivers a range of interventions which achieve the best possible outcomes for patients. As discussed in Chapter 4, in addition to the work it undertakes within its own confines, the PDU also has the potential to function as a kind of catalyst to bring together the work of the many different professions and departments across the organisation, in order to achieve this. The provision of quality care and treatment depend on all professions working together with patients. No single profession can work alone. Failure to recognise these apparently simple truths can only result in less effective service which does not serve patients well.

The PDU also acts as somewhere to try out new ideas in a real clinical setting. This provides a trust with an excellent way of testing innovatory approaches where staff are willing to 'have a go' and where proper evaluation can be conducted. Whenever there was some new initiative such as resource management, reprofiling, using 'syndicate' student nurses to develop protocols, developing links with European hospitals, the PDU was there to say 'we'll try that'.

Having a development unit within a trust can do much to raise its profile. In the case of Seacroft, the hospital was not part of a Trust when the PDU was established, but was directly managed by the local health authority. Being a small hospital, Seacroft was very much in the shadow of the much larger and more widely known university hospitals in Leeds. The PDU was quite successful at publicising itself around the region, through conferences, publications, nursing networks, links with universities and so on. There has been a fairly constant stream of visitors to the unit, usually interested in seeking development unit status for themselves. Such attention has the obvious benefit of creating great pride amongst staff in their work, as they explain their achievements to others. This did much to motivate everyone through a period of three to four years when there was a phenomenal amount of change at Seacroft as it 'changed hands' with other hospitals several times. The merger of Seacroft with the St James's Trust was to provide the greatest challenge yet, the implications of which are discussed further in Chapter 12.

The benefit which is of increasing importance is the PDU's research profile. As part of a university hospital trust, the amount of research activity is important in determining in part how much funding is allocated to the trust. The national Research Assessment Exercise awards points to university research departments on the basis of the quantity and quality of research. Although the PDU did not count as an academic department, in its small way it is able to contribute to the overall research profile of the Trust. In addition, the emphasis upon multidisciplinary research activity fits well with the requirements for collaborative research proposals demanded increasingly by funding bodies.

Recent trends

There has been a trend for NDUs to start calling themselves PDUs, although what is meant by the term seems to vary. The reasons for this are not clear. Whether this represents a change in name only or a more fundamental shift in philosophy only time will tell. Within the Northern and Yorkshire region there has much been discussion between Seacroft PDU and the accreditation team at the Centre for the Development of Nursing Policy and Practice (formerly the Institute of Nursing) at Leeds University. Seacroft has actively tried to influence the accreditation process so as to encourage a more multidisciplinary dimension to the assessment of aspiring development units. It may be that the arguments are beginning to have an impact. Also the many visits to Seacroft provided an opportunity to explain the PDU philosophy first hand. Whatever the reason, it is encouraging that nurses are thinking more broadly about how nursing contributes to the team effort.

Conclusion

The Seacroft PDU has much in common with NDUs and owes much to the ideas and inspiration generated by them. There is a shared concern with quality of care, with the involvement of patients in decision making, with a desire to develop practice to better serve the needs of patients, and to base practice on sound research evidence. Where the PDU differs from NDUs is with the emphasis on multidisciplinary working as a means to better patient care, rather than the development of a single profession as an end in itself. Both approaches have been productive however, and there is no 'right' model. Practitioners must look to their local circumstances and decide what is most appropriate for them. There is also a general message for managers about how much more thought and attention needs to be given to getting the best out of their staff. The organisational culture of some large trusts is stifling ideas and initiative. Such a failure to capitalise on the energy and enthusiasm of staff committed to the best in patients' care is at best a waste of skills and at worst is actually damaging patient care by not addressing serious problems of inefficiency and ineffectiveness.

Part II
The PDU in practice

Chapter 6
Multidisciplinary innovation

David Allsopp

In this chapter three projects are discussed which provide an illustration of how the PDU supported innovative approaches to problems.

- The first, Dealing Decently with Death, arose out of the need to tackle problems related to death in hospital.
- The second concerned the assessment of patient nutritional status and the use of audit to evaluate how well the hospital dealt with the nutritional needs of patients.
- The third describes how PDU staff developed a multidisciplinary patient assessment process and introduced documents to assist both this and the discharge planning process.

All serve to show how the multidisciplinary philosophy worked in practice. Successes and obstacles to progress are discussed and lessons are highlighted. Before the projects are discussed, explanation is first of all needed of what is meant by 'innovation' in the context of the PDU. The links between innovation, creativity and change are discussed, and some of the influences on PDU thinking are presented.

Innovation, creativity, participation and change

The PDU philosophy specifically states that

> The PDU is a centre for innovative, creative practice where change for the better is accepted as an essential feature of development.

The ideas of innovation and creativity are often linked, as creativity is seen as part of the process of inventing new things. The concern is not so much with inventing new technologies but with inventing new processes, new solutions, new systems. Rickards (1985) writes of innovation as 'a process whereby new ideas are put into practice.' The need is for staff to be innovative in trying new approaches to practice, to 'create' new ways of looking at problems and dealing with them. It was realised in the PDU that senior staff did not and could not have all the answers. Sometimes they did not even understand the problems, which were often related to aspects of clinical practice from which more senior staff are relatively remote. Old solutions to problems would not necessarily serve well in the future. New and more flexible ways of dealing with problems were needed. There was also a need to be more proactive than reactive, trying to anticipate problems before they became too large to deal with effectively. As has been stressed in earlier chapters, the PDU emphasised a multidisciplinary approach to usually complex problems faced in providing quality patient care. In other words, care and treatment are more effectively delivered by a multidisciplinary team working well together, understanding and respecting each other's roles, with efficient and effective communication and with a focus on the needs of patients.

Changes such as these represent a major shift, not only in NHS culture but in the way in which organisations of all types are having to respond to increasingly competitive environments. It is beyond the scope of this book to analyse in any depth the reasons for such changes in the NHS. Certainly part of the explanation lies in the introduction of general management, which has encouraged a wider diversity of thinking about ways of delivering quality services; as health care becomes more complex and technological, it becomes necessary to rely on professionals to form their own judgements about how to treat patients within a framework of guidelines rather than rigid prescription.

Some managers have developed ideas about participatory management styles independently. Others will have been influenced by the work of management writers such as Peters and Waterman (1982), who found that innovation was often more closely associated with leadership styles which are participative and collaborative. Whether the findings of a study of American corporations is applicable to a public sector health service in the UK is debatable. However, changes in NHS organisational structures, with the loss of middle layers of management and the consequent devolution of responsibility downwards, have also been a factor influencing the change of culture. The need for greater flexibility and the rapid pace of change meant that those closer to problems would have to be more involved in solving them.

In the PDU this meant trying to release the enormous amount of energy amongst staff; to encourage them to put more in and get more out of their jobs. No extra resources were available. Any new developments had to be generated from the efforts of staff.

The PDU provides a way of overturning a hierarchical hospital system so as to make it more democratic and egalitarian, encouraging everyone to feel that they could suggest new ways of doing things. What matters is the quality of an idea, not who thought of it. The desire was for an open, democratic unit which recognised the contributions of all, not just those at the top, so that a nursing auxiliary could quite safely challenge a consultant over some issue of practice without being shouted at. It was asking a lot.

It was important to allow a certain amount of well-considered risk taking. This was necessary because until something is tested, no one really knows if it will work. What is vital is that serious thought is given to what could go wrong, and mistakes avoided as far as possible. The wider the consultation process, the more that relevant staff are involved in planning, the less likely things can go wrong.

One of the difficulties the PDU sought to overcome was that the NHS did not generally have a culture which encouraged staff to participate in seeking to improve practice. Trying to overturn several decades of NHS culture which had positively discouraged all of these things was a major task. A fiercely hierarchical structure with layers of bureaucracy was not the best way of promoting innovation and development.

The research of social psychologists West and Farr (1990) into innovation at work identified some common features of groups which introduced innovations successfully. These are vision, participative safety, concerns with excellence in quality of task performance, and support for innovation. These ideas were an important influence on the thinking of those involved in setting up the PDU and are now discussed.

Vision

People at work can be motivated by some valued outcome or higher order goal. Groups are more effective if they have clearly identified objectives, and motivation is increased if the objectives are valued by the group. In the case of the PDU what motivated staff was a commitment to providing quality care for specifically elderly patients and the desire to preserve an effective multidisciplinary team. Shared visions are important, and group members are more likely to be committed to them if they are negotiated rather than imposed. Much of the early work in the PDU focused on agreeing a shared vision through 'time out' sessions involving as many staff as possible.

Participative safety

Staff are positively encouraged to take part in decision making in what must be a non-threatening environment. Such involvement needs to be non-judgemental and supportive, and has been shown to be 'associated with less resistance to change and greater likelihood of innovation' (West and Farr, 1990, p. 312). High levels of participation do not on their own indicate strong group cohesion, since such involvement in decision making may be in the pursuit of factional political goals. What matters for innovation to occur is the level of safety perceived to exist. If proposing an idea leads to personal attack, ridicule or disadvantage this is likely to discourage someone from putting new ideas forward. The PDU worked hard at trying to promote such a safety culture.

Excellence in quality of task performance

West and Farr describe a 'shared concern with excellence of quality of task performance in relation to shared vision or outcomes' (p. 313). In other words, the team wants to do an excellent job, and has systems for evaluating and monitoring performance and emphasises individual and team accountability. Other factors include 'feedback and cooperation; mutual monitoring; appraisal of performance of ideas; clear outcome criteria; exploration of opposing opinions; and a concern to maximise quality of task performance' (p. 314).

In the PDU there was a strong emphasis on evaluation and quality monitoring. The influence of the quality 'movement' in the NHS was a relevant factor, with the arrival of audit in all professions. The PDU was very active in promoting a multidisciplinary approach to audit which encouraged the sharing of audit results between professions in clinical audit meetings attended by all. Any new project was required to have clearly defined objectives to evaluate success and the research practitioner had an important role here in assisting with data gathering, analysis and reporting.

As West and Farr (p. 314) said: 'Commitment to excellence therefore creates a demanding group environment in which new and existing practices are appraised and challenged in a constructive way; high standards of performance are encouraged, and a diversity of approaches to achieving excellence is tolerated'.

Support for innovation

Active support is provided for those wishing to try out new ways of doing things. Such initiative is encouraged. Both articulated and enacted support are necessary for innovation to take place. Rewards for those who propose and introduce new ideas are useful and the PDU tries within limited resources to show approval for such activity. This is usually by giving time to staff to work on projects, by providing study leave and by publicising achievements. Safe experimentation is necessary, with the understanding that any failures must be stopped immediately. For example, there was a period in the PDU when some staff conducted questionnaire surveys of patients without first discussing their plans with anyone. This exposed patients to poor quality and potentially upsetting questions, with little thought to presentation, wording or how the survey would be analysed. Such experiences led to the insistence that all ideas must go through a screening process, by checking with the PDU leader or research practitioner at an early stage. The research advisory group was also part of this process.

Innovation as a multidisciplinary activity

As explained in Chapter 5, the major difference between a PDU and an NDU is the emphasis on multidisciplinary working in the PDU. This is partly about encouraging collaborative approaches which enhance the effectiveness of the team, but it is also about asking the team to be innovative in the way they work together. The focus is on the interfaces between professions and means at times asking difficult questions about who does what. Such issues are a necessary part of the debate about the professional status of nursing which is so much of a concern to NDUs. Any discussion about the development of nursing almost inevitably involves other disciplines.

More recent developments in interprofessional education have given strength to the PDU philosophy. The national Centre for the Advancement of Interprofessional Education (CAIPE, established in 1987) in its statement of principles actually says

> the complexities of care cannot be met by the expertise of any one profession in isolation. Collaboration between professionals is necessary to achieve high standards and to respond effectively to the needs and expectations of service users (CAIPE, 1996).

Other CAIPE principles which are consistent with the PDU approach include the involvement of service users and carers, inter-professional collaboration, encouraging professions to learn from each other, respect for the integrity and contributions of each profession and increased professional satisfaction. Similarly, the first recommendation of the report *In the Patient's Interest* (DOH, 1996b) stated

> all professionals in the health and social services should adopt a collaborative approach to working across organisational boundaries, so that patients and their informal carers receive help which is timely, well coordinated, effective and appropriate to their needs.

Examples of such collaboration now follow.

Dealing Decently with Death

The Dealing Decently with Death project was set up initially as part of a hospital-wide quality initiative to tackle various problems which had been addressed separately, or not at all. Some were more serious and pressing than others, but all were relevant to the process of dealing with death in hospital. Some issues arose because of a failure to observe policies whilst others had come to the attention of the project group when they began to explore the problems. Generally speaking, a significant proportion of complaints to hospitals are concerned with the way death is dealt with. It is vitally important that these issues are handled properly and sensitively.

The aims of the project were to identify problems in the current process following the death of a patient in order to improve that process for bereaved relatives and friends.

The issues included:

* the preparation of bodies before transfer from ward to mortuary
* body viewing policy
* support for relatives and friends of the deceased
* support for staff following a death
* the administration side of death in hospital (including the signing and processing of death certificates).
* organ donation was also identified as a relevant issue but it was decided to tackle this separately.

The project group included nurses, the PDU leader, clergy, portering staff, the infection control nurse, medical records staff, therapy managers, a social worker and mortuary staff. It was helpful to have a hospital director-level person on the group as a way of showing senior management commitment to the project. There was also input from the Macmillan nurse, the bereavement liaison officer and the domestic services contractor. Doctors (at senior house officer level) were also invited and did contribute to the work of the group. There are often difficulties involving doctors in practice development. The reasons for this are partly due to practical obstacles like always being 'on call', so that they can be called away from meetings. Also, their six month contracts as junior doctors makes anything other than fleeting involvement in projects very difficult.

It was thought necessary to involve such a wide range of people because of the complex nature of the issues and their interconnectedness. The success of the project depended on the contribution of all involved in the various processes at issue. This was a perfect example of a truly multidisciplinary issue.

The project was led by the PDU leader, who chaired the main group and fed back to a hospital-wide quality improvement group, of which he was a member. Meetings took place as often as twice a month. Several sub-groups were established to focus on specific issues. These met at various intervals depending on the amount and urgency of the work to be done. Work was shared out by asking for volunteers to tackle particular issues. Usually, these volunteers opted for work related to their special expertise.

The fact that the project was set up as a hospital initiative and not a PDU one is an illustration of how the PDU often took the lead and how it dealt with issues of dissemination. It would not have been effective to tackle these issues on the PDU alone. By definition the project was hospital wide and multidisciplinary. Success depended on the involvement of a wide range of people across many departments. It is argued here that the PDU way of working was influential in the way Dealing Decently with Death was approached. The role of the PDU leader was a key factor here, with the leader acting as group facilitator and bringing to the project the values of cooperation, mutual respect, willingness to listen to others' views and to work as a team.

The group began by mapping out the current processes within the hospital related to the deceased patients and their families, and then used these maps to identify specific problems and who should be involved in their resolution. These problems were then translated into clearly stated project objectives. Early successes included the introduction of an audit of last offices practice in response to specific practical problems, and feedback of the results to the ward staff. Nurses on the wards had been previously unaware of the existence of any deficits in their practice or of their consequences for mortuary staff or relatives wishing to view, and this simple exercise resulted very quickly in a significant reduction in reported problems. A second area of development included the identification of delays in the administrative process, which affected the relatives of the deceased. This arose from the difficulty experienced by doctors in completing the death certificate by the necessary deadline. Small changes were made to the existing system to make the process easier for doctors to fit into their other commitments, and additional guidance for new doctors about the correct procedure and the consequences of not achieving a timely completion of the document, was introduced as part of the induction programme.

In spite of these early successes, the nature and complexity of the issues meant it took a long time to work through some of the problems. Nearly two years after the project started, some issues were still unresolved. This was not for want of effort by project participants, but was in part due to the added complication of the hospital merging into another trust with different policies and practices. Work on some of the issues had already been addressed separately in the other trust, and difficulties there had implications for the work on the Seacroft project. In addition, the hospital-wide quality improvement programme of which the Dealing Decently with Death project had been a part (and the supporting framework for this activity) had effectively been phased out at the time of the merger, leaving the project to some extent floating.

The bereavement booklet

There was a need for an information booklet for bereaved relatives which included guidance on what to do following a death. The content of this booklet was developed by members of the project team. However, the only way that could be found to pay for the printing of such a booklet was to include advertisements in it. The income from advertisers would cover the cost, and the revenue would also go into a trust fund to provide bereavement support to staff.

Of course the project group realised the sensitivity surrounding the use of advertisements and devoted considerable discussion to this thorny issue. Amongst the questions debated were whether funeral directors should be invited to advertise, and if so, what form should the adverts take and where should they appear in the booklet. Should there be some constraint on the wording used and if so what?

These issues were debated and resolved within the hospital itself. However, it was at this point that the hospital merged with the much larger teaching hospital. What happened next illustrated how projects can be affected not just by real obstacles, but by perceived ones too. A bereavement booklet had also been produced in the other hospital, and there had been some concerns there about the use of some advertisements. Somehow this developed into a perception that there was a blanket ban on bereavement booklets, a somewhat frustrating outcome after all the work that had been done. In the end the problems were not as great as at first thought, although delays had then been created while everything was unpicked. A booklet for the whole trust was finally agreed and went to the printers.

Bereavement support group for relatives

The project group wanted to set up a bereavement support group for relatives. This was felt to be something which could be done after the booklet was available.

Support for staff

Another aspect of the work involved the establishment of a system of staff support following the death of a patient. This included a staff resource file to be available on each ward and a programme of staff education around bereavement and the hospital's policies for dealing with death. Much of the work was already completed by the project team, but its publication was planned to follow completion of the remainder of the planned project work.

Project group dynamics

The project group worked well together and put in a lot of effort, both at work and in their own time. The whole process of discussing issues that all had a concern with, if from a different angle, was tremendously useful in helping each to understand the others' roles and to appreciate the complex workings of the process of dealing with death in hospital. Staff became aware of problems others were experiencing that they had been unaware of previously. There was also the considerable advantage that those not directly concerned with a problem could see it from a more detached viewpoint and were able to suggest possible solutions which had not occurred to those in the thick of things.

What was perhaps most innovative about the group was the way in which the project brought in new grades of staff. There were some who had never had the experience of being involved in a project such as this. No one had ever asked them to express a view, let alone suggest solutions. This was the PDU at its best, involving staff because they were relevant to a problem, not just because they were senior people. What mattered was the quality of the idea, not who suggested it. Involving people in this way greatly increases the chances of achieving lasting change, by promoting ownership of the problem and the solutions. Making change in this way does a great deal to encourage respect for colleagues and understanding of the difficulties faced.

It was not all plain sailing, however, with some members feeling defensive, as if they were being blamed for problems. This perhaps is one of the stiffest challenges in achieving change. To be able to discuss an issue dispassionately without it being seen as a personal attack requires a certain level of sensitivity and maturity of all concerned. It is a process of learning how to focus on the issue rather than the personality. The tone and example set by group leaders is crucial here.

There were some difficulties for some staff in attending meetings, which lessened the contribution they were able to make, and this meant that those who were regular attenders sometimes carried a disproportionate workload. This does not mean staff were uncommitted to the project, but often the practical difficulties of fixing mutually convenient meetings meant that on occasion 'sub-group' gatherings of only two or three people took place. Others contributed to meetings by post.

This highlights some of the problems in devolving decision making downwards in this way. Staff are expected to find the time to carry on with their jobs at the same time as working on projects that may take them away from their work. At the end of the day practice development using such an approach depends on the willingness not only of those working on projects, but on their colleagues who show their support by covering absences. It truly has to be a team effort.

The ways in which group members felt able to contribute included the supply of information, the identification of aims, leading sub-groups, recording minutes, inviting other relevant people, discussing issues, drafting the bereavement booklet. For some these were new experiences and their involvement enabled them to grow both professionally and personally. New skills were acquired and others developed.

Support for the work of the group

All group members supported each other in working on the project, although it was felt by some that more support from the senior manager acting as project sponsor would have helped get the bereavement booklet completed and in use much earlier. It was very frustrating for some that all the effort put in to consulting widely about the booklet did not come to fruition for many months. One group member commented on this that it was 'very disheartening and does not encourage us to work on similar schemes in future.'

Other forms of support such as clerical support were absent. Notes of meetings were written up and circulated personally by the PDU leader, who also arranged meetings and venues.

Authority of the project group

The group was established to make changes, not just to make recommendations. Its authority was derived from its membership, all of whom had expert knowledge about different aspects of the process of dealing with death in hospital. It was also felt that members had the necessary range of skills both to analyse the problems and to make changes. Some had been through service improvement training courses run by the hospital which taught data collection and analysis, change management and other related skills, but not until after they had become involved in the group.

The group also had management support in the hospital. Difficulties arose when the merger with another hospital took place. This meant in effect that the authority of the group had to be renegotiated. This does not mean to say that the commitment to dealing with the issues was no longer there, but different groups of staff had been working separately on similar issues. To get agreement across the newly merged trust was a complicated new challenge which inevitably delayed progress on the work.

Another factor in the delay was the departure at a key time of the PDU leader, who was an influential member of the group. Although there was only a gap of around six weeks between his departure and the new post holder arriving, this meant that the work lost momentum. It was understandable that the new PDU leader needed time to settle in and it was several months before the project was back on track.

Benefits of involvement in the project

Apart from the changes which the group achieved in Dealing Decently with Death, there were several benefits for participants in terms of their own development. For some it was their first experience of being involved in work like this. Having the opportunity of bringing your own expertise to a discussion of a problem and having a say on the solutions was an invaluable boost to self-esteem, confidence and morale. The skills acquired through involvement in the project were transferable to other situations. The issue of dissemination about which development units worry so much was just as much about the transfer of ideas, values, knowledge and skills as about the products of a project.

Involvement in the project did much to develop participants' teamwork and cooperation skills, their communication and time management skills, their awareness of organisational functioning and decision-making processes, of others' roles and of the effects of decisions on other parts of the organisation. The sense of empowerment whilst on the project was great, although this feeling was for some a little diluted when the project dragged on into its second year.

Some went on to work on other projects, others took their newly found skills back to their wards or departments. All will have grown in the process. All will have become empowered to a greater or lesser extent to influence other decisions and to assert themselves both personally and professionally.

Lessons learned from the project

Perhaps one of the most difficult lessons was the appreciation that some changes can take an awfully long time to achieve. It can take a tremendous amount of energy, perseverance and determination to see something through to its completion. The more that time passes, the more likely it seems that other changes, such as those to do with organisational structures, can influence the success of a project. If the project is itself about changing those structures or the processes associated with them, then the urgency of the task becomes clear. Some problems cannot be solved overnight. Inevitably, the ground is constantly shifting and it takes someone with particularly astute political skills to manoeuvre a course through the minefield. The problems raised by the trust merger might have been foreseen, but it is hard to see what could have been done to avoid them. All that could have been anticipated (as it had been) was that the merger with such a large organisation with a very different culture would provide new challenges to be overcome.

Another lesson learned concerns the difference between a time-limited, quality improvement project group established to tackle specific problems, and everyday operational management functions. Once it was established, there was a tendency to shunt onto the group any issues related to 'death', even though these might fall squarely into specific management functions and could more appropriately have been dealt with there. This perhaps demonstrated a lack of understanding in the wider organisation about the role of such groups and their interface with existing structures. In particular this resulted in difficulties where financial arrangements were involved.

Nutrition assessment audit

The work done on nutrition was driven by a Senior Dietitian, Lynn George, who knew from her knowledge of the literature that malnutrition was common in hospital patients, particularly the elderly, and was a problem often missed. It was important to assess the extent to which patients were at risk of developing malnutrition in the PDU. The next task was to find out what nutritional assessment was already being conducted by medical and nursing staff and how many at risk patients were being referred to the dietetics department.

The nutrition audit was led by Lynn, with the support of the Clinical Director who showed a keen interest in the work. Nurses helped with weighing and measuring heights of patients, and the PDU leader and Research Practitioner were also supportive.

The results of the audit confirmed Lynn's fears: that patients in need of dietetic referral and support were not always getting it. In fact, only 58% of patients needing dietetic advice were being referred.

The results were presented at a medical audit meeting and at the clinical meeting held once a week (later to become the Clinical Forum). A report was also circulated to the Clinical Director and Service Manager. The discussions that followed led to the conclusion that patients should be routinely assessed by nurses on admission to hospital. In particular a patient's weight, height and body mass index should inform the decision over referral to the dietitian. Other needs such as special diets were also relevant. These factors were to be built in to the admission assessment document which is discussed later.

Raising the profile of nutrition issues in this way did much to improve rates of referral to the dietitians. Audits were repeated which showed better results each time.

Factors helping success

The success of the change was largely due to the efforts of the dietetic team in gathering evidence of the extent of the problems and in educating staff about the need to consider expert advice. Other factors in supporting the changes included the enthusiasm of other key members of staff including consultants, the PDU leader, research practitioner, service manager and ward managers. There was also a willingness amongst most nursing staff to accept responsibility for nutritional assessment.

Factors inhibiting success

One of the difficulties of implementing change of this sort was that there were so many people to influence. This was not just a PDU issue, it related to all the medical wards in the department. Around 150 nurses had to change their practice. Although various meetings were held, it was often difficult for nurses to attend. Inevitably there were some who were more resistant to the proposals, and their disinterest showed. These were, however, atypical. For the most part, nurses and dietitians worked well together in seeing the changes through. Dietitians relied heavily upon nurses to assess patients, to carry out dietetic advice and to feed patients where necessary. Priorities did not always coincide, but sufficient numbers of nurses appreciated the need for proper nutritional assessment to make the change stick.

The contribution to the development of multidisciplinary teamwork

One of the benefits of different professions working together on a project is that it provides opportunities to explain and promote roles within the team. Teams function much less effectively when members are unclear what others are there for. The nutrition audit work provided a focus for discussion for nurses and dietitians which assisted such understanding. The challenge for the dietitians was to influence members of another discipline to cooperate with their proposals for change. They would only be successful if they could persuade sufficient numbers of nurses of the value of completing patient assessments to make the new system work. What also helped were the changes made to nursing documentation, in which a section on nutrition assessment was included with clear referral criteria to guide nurses.

Dissemination

The work on nutrition assessment demonstrates one of the ways the PDU deals with the issue of dissemination. Rather than pilot the original work in a small area and then seek to spread the ideas further afield, key staff from outside the PDU are involved right from the start. That way they are much more committed to the project and can then act as 'product champions' in their own areas. This approach was one used consistently by the PDU on all sorts of work. It did not always work; it assumes that the people you involve in a project have the necessary skills to implement change and this was not always the case.

Multidisciplinary patient assessment

The work on nutrition led to the other main piece of work undertaken in the PDU – the development of a multidisciplinary patient assessment document.

One of the features of professional practice is the need to keep accurate and timely records so as to provide a legal record and to support communication, usually between members of the same profession. Occasionally, members of other professions will read your records, particularly if you are a doctor. It is perhaps less common for professionals to read records outside their own discipline. For example, in general, nurses will not often read physiotherapy records, nor will doctors read occupational therapy notes. This may be because records are stored in another department. Even less likely is that professions will combine their records into one document. This is usually explained for all sorts of practical reasons, such as the need to have access to records in one's own department for dealing with enquiries after discharge, or because of fears about notes going missing, or where they should be stored. There is also something about having your own professional records as a symbol of professional independence. To merge records may be perceived as an erosion of this, so it is perhaps understandable when resistance to such mergers is expressed.

It was never a PDU aim to combine professional records, but there did seem to be some merit in encouraging staff to use their records to improve communication with each other, both in terms of the referral process and in care planning. All too often groups of professionals believed by their members to be 'teams' are just a collection of people setting goals for (not with) patients. These goals are not always team goals. The extent of coordination will vary from team to team and will depend on all sorts of factors including leadership, effective communication and opportunities to discuss team goals such as care planning meetings.

One of the features of the PDU was the strong multidisciplinary ethos, born out of its history as a service for the elderly. It had always been common practice for teams to meet regularly to discuss the progress of patients and their needs prior to and after discharge. However, it was realised that the increasing trend towards shorter hospital stays with care at home after discharge highlighted various needs: a thorough assessment of patients; better guidance for patients on discharge; better communication between professionals in hospital and those providing community services (Williams *et al.*, 1994). In addition, anything that could reduce the duplication of effort in writing records would be warmly welcomed by all.

In true PDU style, a multidisciplinary project group was set up to develop a new document to replace the traditional nursing 'Kardex'. The fact that nursing notes were kept at the bedside made them the obvious choice in creating a document which all the team could use. The first thing the project group did was to look at the strengths, weaknesses, opportunities and threats (SWOT) of the current approach to professional record keeping.

The SWOT analysis is a very constructive way of getting a project going. It helps all involved to agree on what the issues are. Without such agreement it is difficult to proceed. It also helps staff to realise the positive aspects of their work. This is something not always appreciated. Again, it assists understanding of each other's roles, and it is also rewarding to hear from other professions what they like about your work. This balances any discussion of negative issues, and the attention to opportunities encourages a more positive outlook than a mere concentration on problems. Looking at threats injects necessary realism into the debate, especially about resource issues.

The strengths of having separate professional records were that each profession felt they 'owned' notes which related to their own input, access was easy and use of professional abbreviations saved writing time. The system of written referrals to therapists from doctors satisfied the requirements of professional bodies and professional indemnity insurance.

Having separate records resulted in a fragmented system, with the same information being recorded in duplicate by different professionals in different places. The only part of the record patients had easy access to was the nursing care plan, kept at the bedside. The use of professionally unique abbreviations may have been an advantage within disciplines, but did nothing for interdisciplinary understanding and communication. The referral process could sometimes be delayed, due to the need for a doctor's signature on a referral form. It was more often nurses who initiated the referral in effect, by asking doctors to sign the form. Primary nurses felt an element of frustration at not being able to refer on their own initiative, this being a restriction on their growing sense of autonomy. The 24 hour presence of nurses at the bedside meant they had more opportunities to assess patients' changing needs than those whose presence was confined to 'office hours'. Thus it may have been possible that necessary referrals were missed or delayed.

The review of professional record keeping presented opportunities to promote better understanding of roles, sharing of knowledge and improvements in communication resulting in a more consistent approach to rehabilitation seven days a week. Duplication could be reduced, and a model of assessment based on a collaborative and interdisciplinary framework developed. There was also a need to think much more deeply about how to involve patients and their relatives in the care planning process. One requirement is that professional documentation is easily accessible to them, is clear and easily understood. Finally, there was also a wonderful opportunity to improve the discharge planning process.

Threats to the project included concerns about imparting 'trade secrets' and losing role uniqueness, the potential conflict with guidance from professional bodies which required referrals from doctors, the need for resources to develop and have printed a new patient assessment booklet and the scarcity of time needed to develop the new document (this is a particular problem for therapists, being relatively few in number, and being asked to help out with all sorts of projects). There were also fears about losing the new booklet and about the potential difficulties of trying to involve some patients in decisions about their care.

The process of change

The multidisciplinary group working on the new documentation met regularly over a four month period, during which agreement was reached on several 'trigger factors' for referral. These were built in to an assessment booklet to be used by nurses when admitting a patient to a ward. The plan was that nurses would be able to bring in a physiotherapist, occupational therapist or other professional if a patient met the criteria set out in the booklet (this process did not include referrals by doctors to other medical specialities, which continued in the normal way). The therapist, on receiving a referral, would then assess the patient's needs and then treat as they saw fit. Referrals could be made by phone or by direct request as the therapist visited the ward. It was expected that this would speed up the referral process, enabling patients to be assessed more quickly and treatment started earlier.

As far as possible, the booklet incorporated validated and well known assessment scales such as Barthel for functional ability, Waterlow for pressure sore risk, the Glasgow coma scale and a pain assessment scale. It was possible to use these scales or parts of them for the referral trigger factors. For example, the Barthel Index could also be used to assess need for physiotherapy and occupational therapy input. A Body Mass Index score, with other information, could form the basis of a referral to dietitians. Where valid scales did not exist, a few simple direct questions could assess the need for referral to others such as the speech and language therapist. The need for social work referral was linked to the process of complex assessment by social services as part of the requirements of the Community Care Act. In addition, the Waterlow score helped the process of deciding on pressure relieving aids, and had the added benefit of being the scale used by community nurses.

As well as assessment information, the booklet also included a discharge letter designed to be given to the patient, with details on medication, aids and adaptations, outpatient appointments, a teaching care plan and contact phone numbers for the primary nurse, dietitian and pharmacy helpline.

Once the content of the assessment booklet had been agreed, the next problem was how to pay for a print run. Fortunately, the Regional Heath Authority were inviting bids for their Small Grants Scheme and the PDU was successful in getting necessary funds.

The next step was to pilot the new booklet on two PDU wards. It was important to evaluate the results of the pilot, and there were several issues: the appropriateness of referrals made by nurses; the extent of use of parts of the booklet; the value of the booklet in improving communication. Dietetic colleagues were also keen to know if using the booklet improved the nutritional status of patients.

Referral criteria

Referral to dietitians could only come from medical (or dental) practitioners (this was related to the dietetic code of practice). It was therefore agreed that a blanket referral system would be put in place. This enabled nurses to refer without having to seek the signature of a doctor on each occasion.

The audits demonstrated improved referral rates and showed that nurses were recording more useful information than before, and compared with non-PDU wards. They were also becoming more adept at using this information in care plans. The nutrition audit showed that nurses were conducting a much more comprehensive assessment of nutritional needs of patients and that referral rates had increased significantly. All of this helped to improve communication between disciplines.

As well as the assessment booklet, communication was improved by the use of care planning sheets which anyone in the team could use (examples can be seen in Faulkner, 1996). In addition to the nursing care plan, physiotherapists and occupational therapists would write what they were doing so that a much more comprehensive picture of overall care could be seen together. This was particularly of benefit to patients, who had ready access to care plans at the bedside and were encouraged to read them. For the therapists, adding to the care plan was duplicating what they already wrote in their own records, which they wished to maintain separately.

After a year or so of using the assessment booklet, it was decided that it was in need of review. One problem was its A5 size, which was too small, and the attempt at covering all the needs for assessment made it too unwieldy, especially for short stay patients with simple needs. It was agreed that two booklets would be developed, both A4 size. The first was intended for the initial assessment of most patients. It included less detail, but enabled basic information to be recorded, and included the trigger factors for referral. If a patient was admitted with more complex needs, or became more dependent, the second booklet could be used. Some alterations to detail were made, but the content remained largely the same.

Further changes were to follow, with the realisation that nurses had a tendency to use the simpler initial assessment booklet, even when the more comprehensive document was appropriate. This was because it saved time. Another reason for change was the desire to rationalise data recording. When patients were admitted to the department, they were asked for their biographical details (name, address, next-of-kin etc.) no less than three times. The plan was to integrate the reception unit clinical assessment form used by nurses there, with the admission sheet required by the patient administration department, and the ward assessment booklet. This was no mean task.

Again, a multidisciplinary group was established, including patient administration staff. From the start of the review to delivery of the new documents took 18 months. This was due to the scale of the exercise, as this review sought to adapt the documents equally for use in all specialties across the hospital. There were also difficulties in finding funds to pay for initial print runs. Although it would have been possible to use photocopies, experience had shown that even if the quality of these is good to start with, they soon deteriorate. It also means that some member of the hospital staff spends wasteful time doing the copying. It is far better to have professionally printed documents.

Discharge planning

At the same time as the assessment booklet was being developed, the issue of patient discharge planning was becoming a prominent issue. Here was something which was at the very heart of multidisciplinary working. Effective discharge planning was all about a needs-led approach involving the patient and family, about clarity of team roles and aims, about speedy and effective communication and inter-agency collaboration. The PDU prided itself on the way in which it provided a model for effective discharge planning. The introduction in the PDU of the multidisciplinary patient assessment document coincided with changes brought about by the Community Care Act in 1991. This required a comprehensive assessment process, led by social services, by which patients' needs for placement after discharge were to be judged. The work done in the PDU in developing the assessment document helped a great deal in preparing staff from all disciplines for the changes brought about by the act. Much of the information required under the comprehensive assessment process was already collected in the PDU and it was therefore fairly straight-forward for staff to adapt to the new system. A discharge planning checklist was already incorporated into the assessment document, with copies for the patient of information on diagnosis, treatment and follow up. Later, the idea for a discharge planning document which provided information useful to patient and carer, with carbon copies for the patient's records, the GP and community nurse was produced. This very quickly turned out to be totally unwieldy, and had to be abandoned in favour of a much simpler document.

The process of discharge planning increasingly became a hot political issue, as patients waiting for discharge experienced delays due to the difficulties social services had in funding sufficient nursing and residential home placements. The trust employed a nurse to act as discharge planning coordinator for the medical division, and at the same time a new community liaison nurse was appointed. This provided fresh impetus to the process. The community liaison nurse was based part time in the PDU and on appointment was supported in settling in by the PDU leader. Through these roles the PDU was increasingly beginning to have an influence city wide.

Lessons learned

The lessons learned from all this are that it can take a long time to implement change, particularly where a unit like the PDU is seeking to influence outside its own confines as well as within, and determination and perseverance are needed. Also, it seems one can go on for ever trying to improve documentation, and even then, never satisfy everyone. There will always be someone who wants something added, or taken out, or a box bigger or smaller. There comes a point when you have to jump and live with what you have created. The booklets always attracted attention whenever we presented them at conferences or study days. People were always asking for copies, which seems to suggest that reviewing documentation is common practice. It seems that everyone wants documentation tailor-made to their local needs. There needs to be a compromise between those needs and the costs. In the end, the successful recording of quality information about patients depends as much on the person using it as on the design of the form. A lot can be done to make it more likely that certain information is recorded, like asking the right questions and by giving people enough room to write in. There was an obvious concern about the possibility of nurses recording data not relevant to their own practice. However, given the nature of the clinical work undertaken in the PDU, all the data collected were relevant to nurses and could be used directly in the writing of nursing care plans.

Conclusion

The projects discussed have illustrated practical ways in which the PDU works. It has not all been plain sailing, but much can be learned even when things do not always go according to plan. What is vitally important is that attempts are made to improve things for patients which involve all relevant people. Failure to do this will limit the extent of success.

Chapter 7
Research and the Practice Development Unit

David Allsopp

Why is research important to the PDU?

During the early discussions about setting up the PDU one of the questions repeatedly asked was what would make a PDU different from any well run ward? All the emphasis upon innovation, quality care and effective team working could equally well apply anywhere. The only thing that most clinical areas did not do was research. Those that did seemed to have a higher profile, although the research was commonly led by doctors, whose research interests were either concerned with laboratory work or with clinical trials. Research units were usually part of a university department. NDUs were also keen to promote research-based practice. Alan Pearson, in his study of the Burford NDU, declared that one of the aims was to find out if 'the changes currently being advocated by nursing's academic elite be implemented in an "ordinary" unit' (Pearson, 1992).

So research became a principal aim. It was not expected that everyone should do research; most would not, although all professionals should be able to read and make sense of straightforward research publications and know how to apply them to practice. It is interesting that much of this thinking foreshadowed the more recent national initiatives on clinical effectiveness. The PDU sought to bring research findings closer to clinical practice right from the start.

There were other benefits besides raising the profile of the unit. It was felt that by having some staff actually doing research in the department this would help to promote the questioning culture which was thought to be necessary to developing practice. Staff needed to critically examine their practice, and this process had been assisted considerably by the audit work done in the hospital. By doing research it was hoped that opportunities to learn and develop new skills would be provided, that this would provide a stimulating work environment which in turn would motivate staff and assist recruitment and retention. These ideas will now be discussed in more depth.

The role of research and audit in developing a questioning culture

Both audit and research have a role in developing practitioners to think critically about their practice. Both are valuable in requiring that evidence is considered systematically. The PDU placed a particular emphasis upon evaluation of project work and felt that this was important enough to appoint a research practitioner to promote a research culture and support work on evaluation. It was important that research was shown to be something that could be done by professionals other than doctors, not just by academics in their ivory towers or by nurses working on someone else's drug trial. Not that these are not important too, but these approaches seemed to perpetuate the idea that research was an elitist thing to do. The aim was for nurses and physiotherapists and occupational therapists and others to have the opportunity to be involved in research, if only in a small way at first. They needed to see that research can be useful, interesting and motivating, and that professional practice could be developed through research.

Closing the theory–practice gap

Another reason for promoting research activity in the PDU was a concern about the so-called theory–practice gap. Very few professionals have direct contact with or get involved in research, which is commonly done by scientists in universities. Such a separation of research and practice was seen as a major obstacle to the implementation of research findings into practice. If professionals never had any contact with research, never got involved or knew what it was about, how could they ever be expected to read and appreciate published research as something valuable to help their practice? There was a need to demystify research and to give people a sense that they too could be instrumental in developing new knowledge about practice.

Audit activity in the PDU

All clinical teams need to think critically about their professional practice and devise new and better ways of treating patients and improving results. Research is not necessary to achieve that. The growing interest in audit was certainly a factor in stimulating a culture that questioned practice. Audit required a change from thinking about the single patient and his or her problems to thinking about aggregate numbers of patients. Audit used some of the techniques of research in terms of data gathering and analysis, although it was less rigorous. In any case, research asks different questions from audit. Research asks questions like 'what is going on here?' or 'what is the best way to treat this problem?' Audit asks 'are we doing it the way the research says we should be?' So there is considerable value in conducting both audit and research. One of the problems of audit is that it is often conducted 'top-down', by some senior nurse or manager, or by a central department. A lot of audit also seems to depend on the written professional record as the main source of evidence that practice takes place in a particular way.

Involving the people who deliver the care in setting the standards to be audited is one way of generating a sense of ownership of the problem and the process. This is an approach used in the PDU from time to time. Whenever possible and appropriate a multidisciplinary approach to standard setting was used. This can be a very valuable way of breaking down barriers between professions and helping to create a better understanding of each other's roles. Some things have to be tackled in a uniprofessional way however. Sometimes professions work separately towards a common goal.

Take stroke audit, for example. A multidisciplinary group was established, led by a dietitian, to develop a stroke audit process to complement the Royal College of Physicians Stroke Audit Package used by the doctors. The group agreed on the elements of the process through which most stroke patients passed during their hospital stay. The professions were then asked to define standards for their particular inputs into the process. These were then to form the basis of the audit. All this took well over a year. One of the difficulties for therapists such as the physiotherapists and occupational therapists is that there are so few of them relative to nurses. Because they get asked to participate in all sorts of groups, committees and other activities, they find it very difficult to find the time for everything.

During this period, the Department of Medicine merged with other directorates into a new medical and elderly division. The issue of dissemination arose, and it seemed sensible to seek to achieve a divisional consensus on the stroke standards. One difficulty here was that the rest of the trust appeared to work in very uniprofessional ways. The idea of agreeing multidisciplinary standards for stroke care did not seem to occur to some, although it seemed obvious to

PDU staff. The first step was to approach nurses in other parts of the Division with interest in stroke nursing and ask if they would be willing to agree on a Divisional standard for stroke nursing care. It seemed easier to do it this way rather than get together a multidisciplinary group to represent the whole Division. This was partly because the therapists were managed within a separate directorate and there were practical difficulties in getting everyone together from different sites across the city, apart from the problems on agreeing something on such a scale. The promotion of close multiprofessional working needs an incredible amount of local support and coordination, done by someone who knows and understands the issues surrounding multidisciplinary politics.

Whilst audit was useful in raising questions about practice, there were some worries at times about the quality of audit activity. Sometimes it seemed as if audit was just bad research. It was particularly worrying when decisions were sometimes taken on the basis of an audit of a very small sample of half-randomly selected case notes or nursing records. Perhaps the fact that people do not often change their practice just because some audit suggests change is a blessing in disguise. What a waste of effort, though.

What audit has achieved is that professions are beginning to talk to each other about practice. Over two or three years, the separate uniprofessional audit arrangements gradually came together. There was a monthly medical audit meeting, at which doctors would present the findings of drug audits, or treatment protocol audits. Every third month this developed into a multidisciplinary clinical audit meeting which included doctors too. Audit topics would as far as possible cover issues of interest to all. These meetings, usually lasting two hours, were excellent since they got everyone in a room together where they had to listen to others talking about their practice. Although it was a fairly informal gathering, there were often some stiff challenges to presentations, and some lively debates! For some, to present at the clinical audit meeting was quite a daunting experience. If possible staff could have a practice run at the weekly clinical forum meeting, where there was usually a smaller and more friendly audience.

The main thing was to get professionals talking about their practice together. The value of this cannot be stressed highly enough as a way of promoting understanding of roles and a team ethic.

Raising the profile of the PDU

In order that the PDU could disseminate the results of its work it was important that the unit was known about. In a sense the unit had to 'sell' its products and needed to present itself so that its work was credible and respected. If the PDU could be seen to be success-fully carrying out quality research, this would add to the unit's credibility and help to raise its profile. Publication of research would help to publicise the PDU and help disseminate ideas and innovations.

With the support of regional NDU networks the PDU was able to make its work known, through conferences and publications. There were a constant stream of visitors who were interested in the PDU and wished to see 'how we did it', some from as far away as Plymouth. Such visits provided an excellent opportunity to spread the multidisciplinary philosophy of the PDU. There remained however the issue of credibility within the Trust. Seacroft's merger with the St James's University Hospitals Trust on 1 April 1995 provided a challenge to prove that the work was worthwhile and should continue.

Opportunities to learn and develop new skills

One of the advantages of working in the PDU was that the emphasis on research provided opportunities for staff to learn and develop new skills in research. The hospital supported nurses doing the post-registration research course (ENB 870) and the PDU encouraged multidisciplinary involvement in research into self-medication and stroke rehabilitation. It is rewarding to see how motivated people become when they do a research course, wanting to do research of their own. The feedback from staff was very positive. They often said how much they realised they had taken for granted before. Doing the research course had forced them to question practice as they never had before. They realised the limits to knowledge about health care and the best ways of dealing with problems patients and practition-ers face.

PDU support for research

Research is a highly skilled activity, sometimes done badly. It takes lots of time and not insubstantial amounts of money. Finding the time and getting hold of research funds is very difficult. The way forward was to establish an infrastructure which would support those wishing to pursue research, and to try to get some funding. There were two main strands to the support provided: a research advisory group (RAG) and the creation of a research practitioner role as a development of the nursing quality assurance role.

Research Advisory Group

The RAG was established early on in the life of the PDU. The purpose was to provide easy access to expert knowledge and advice about research. There were several people around the hospital who had the necessary skills and experience in both qualitative and quantitative approaches to research. Links with the nursing section of the local polytechnic (as it was then) were fruitful, with both a senior and principal lecturer who were very keen to support RAG. In addition, the medical service manager was part of RAG, since it was felt to be important that the resource implications of any research proposal should be considered. The PDU leader and quality assurance nurse also participated, as both had experience of research.

There was a very real commitment to supporting research which addressed issues of a multidisciplinary nature. It was agreed that if RAG could not help with a particular proposal or idea, then it would help identify other possible sources of support.

Terms of reference for RAG were agreed and the group met monthly depending on demand.

Research Advisory Group Terms of Reference

- To provide advice and encouragement to all staff wishing to carry out research
- To support staff in seeking publication of research
- To act as a resource by providing appropriate educational support
- To establish a reputation for supporting and fostering interest in research
- To offer multidisciplinary links
- To review research in progress.

The idea was that any member of PDU staff, whoever they were, would have an idea for some research they wanted to do. The idea could be as vague as 'I want to do some research into pressure sore treatment' or 'I want to find out what it's like to discover you have diabetes', to a well developed proposal bidding for research grant money.

Most people from all the professions had little or no direct experience of research and would not know where to start. In an attempt to foster a spirit of enquiry, PDU staff were encouraged to be free to ask searching questions about their practice and to have some idea of how they might begin to find answers to their questions.

Problems faced by the Research Advisory Group

One of the difficulties was how formidable RAG could appear to a member of staff with no research background and no experience of presenting ideas for research. RAG needed to be as informal as possible. For the first two years or so RAG was quite active in advising staff on various proposals. However, it became increasingly clear that fewer proposals were coming forward and meetings were cancelled as there was little demand for them. This was quite a worrying development, as it seemed to indicate that staff were losing interest in research. What factors explained the growing lack of interest? The most significant was the fact that research was just nowhere near the top of people's agendas in the way that it had been. The pressures on staff due to increasing workload and the uncertainties created by repeated reorganisations took their toll. It was enough of a task to complete the work expected of them without having to think about research as well. On its own the RAG was not enough to stimulate people to come up with ideas. It needed much more active support at ward level to generate the energy and enthusiasm required. The decision in 1996 to declare the whole Department of Medicine a PDU made such support more difficult to provide. There were also other priorities which had to take precedence over research, such as staffing the wards and mandatory training.

Another factor in the decline in interest in the research advisory group was that increasingly staff were going on courses which gave them research skills, such as degrees and ENB courses. What remained important was that staff had support available if they wanted advice on research. Consequently, the Research Support Network was set up with the Research Practitioner as the main link in the Department. Anyone needing advice could be helped directly or put in touch with someone who could help. The Trust's own Research and Development Department could provide statistical advice, and various others could also assist both within the Trust and outside.

The development of a research and development strategy for the hospital

Initially the work done to support research was restricted to the PDU. There was no remit to extend the strategy beyond this to other medical wards or to the surgical or infectious diseases department. However, in practice the arrangement became increasingly flexible.

When it came to establishing the role of research practitioner, it was an obvious time to consider research and development for the whole Seacroft site. The strategy developed was, of course, multidisciplinary. Its goals were to increase the calibre and quantity of research and development activity across the hospital, and to maximise the impact of this work upon the quality and cost effectiveness of patient care.

There were three principal elements to the strategy:

- development of research and development (R&D) infrastructure and support, including a focus on skills development and leadership across the professions
- development of R&D understanding and activity at all levels
- integration of R&D understanding into the broader work of the hospital.

This provided a model of R&D support which involved both 'bottom-up' and hospital level generation of activity, with the benefits of a multidisciplinary practice development unit functioning as a resource to the hospital as a whole, and as a test-bed for new ideas.

Principles underpinning the R&D strategy

There were a number of important principles relevant to the strategy. The first was empowerment – of patients and staff. Staff were empowered by giving them the skills to critically evaluate their practice and to strengthen their professionalism through greater knowledge and skills. A much more patient focused approach to research and development was required, making it possible for patients to play an increasingly direct role in expressing a voice about the service being delivered. That meant exploring new approaches to involvement in decision-making processes, such as in the diabetes project. It meant giving much more serious thought to the idea of involving patients in setting the research agenda. This was much more difficult, and meant asking such questions of patients as 'what research do you think we should be doing?' and 'how do you think we should be doing this research?' The latter question is perhaps the easier of the two. Service users are more likely to be able to say whether they have a preference for interviews, questionnaires or focus groups as a means of finding out what they think, than to say what research should be done. Thinking up research questions is difficult enough even for people who have the right knowledge and skills.

Another important principle was of course a strong multidisciplinary approach. This did not necessarily mean trying to involve everyone in each research project. Where possible and appropriate research should involve some form of multidisciplinary collaboration, and tackle issues of a multidisciplinary nature. There was also a need to think through the multidisciplinary implications of any change sought as a result of the research done.

Research which was relevant to only one profession was not to be excluded, and was both necessary and desirable. It was hoped that medical research would be included in the strategy, and that one day doctors would bring their ideas to RAG and be prepared to discuss them in a multidisciplinary forum. However, doctors often have their own arrangements, usually tied in with career development.

Many in the PDU were new to research and did not fully appreciate the politics of research and its funding. Doctors had for many years been the main recipients of research funding and other professions often found it difficult to gain access. To its credit, Yorkshire Region seemed slowly to be responding to pressures to encourage nurses and others to bid for funds. Getting nurses and others on to the grant awarding committees was part of the solution. By 1996, the establishment of the Nursing Effectiveness Centre at the Centre for Reviews and Dissemination at York University was a significant step.

The research practitioner role

The post of research practitioner was a new one and had evolved out of the role of the quality assurance nurse. When Seacroft merged with the St James's Trust there was a review of the role of the quality assurance nurse at Seacroft and several options were considered. It was decided that the PDU needed to apply more rigour to evaluation since it was important to be able to provide good quality evidence about PDU activity. This required someone with data handling skills and research abilities. Much of the evaluation work would involve data gathering, sometimes by questionnaire survey, sometimes by interview. Data analysis skills were also required, preferably involving qualitative and quantitative methods. Some would argue that audit would be sufficient, and access to the clinical audit department would have given the PDU the support needed. However, publication in refereed professional journals needed more than audit results, it needed research.

Research training

Part of the research practitioner role involved teaching research awareness, not just within the PDU but more widely across the Trust. For two years a research awareness study day was run at Seacroft. Efforts were combined with those of the Trust's Nursing Research and Practice Development Unit to run study days two or three times a year, eligible to anyone in the Trust.

The Trust's Research and Development Department

The merger of Seacroft with the St James's Trust opened up access to support not easily available previously. The Research and Development Department's role was to support bids for research funds and to provide educational support. Through a monthly newsletter they circulated information about pending deadlines for research bids with various funding organisations such as charities or NHS sources. Application forms were easily available, which helped a great deal. Some very good study days were conducted and statistical training courses were free or at low cost to Trust staff. The department's statistician was very helpful to the PDU in providing advice and input to RAG.

Research funding

There had been some early PDU success in bidding for funding from the regional health authority for audit funds under a 'Nursing and Therapy Audit' scheme. Applications for larger research grants had met with no success.

Changes in research funding mechanisms

The Culyer Report (1994) proposed changes in the way research in the NHS was funded so that there was a single funding stream for research. Trusts would bid not for individual projects but for funds to support a package of projects. The implications for the PDU of this new approach were that it would have to compete within the trust to have research proposals included in the trust bid to Region. It was not clear at first how much of a problem this might be. There were some very powerful medical voices in the trust, some of which had many years of research experience and success at gaining grants. How could the PDU possibly hope to compete with such as these? Claims by some that it would all be sewn up by the doctors were resisted by medics who pointed to the shift in attitude at region towards a recognition of the value of supporting research done by non-medics.

The other significant change in Northern and Yorkshire was the abolition of closing dates for applications for funding. This meant that bids could be sent in any time, and would be considered at the next committee meeting, or referred to the subsequent one. This gave more time for the preparation of bids, hopefully improving the quality and likely success rate.

What remained vitally important was that bids for research funds continued. No bid, no success. Bidding also provided priceless experience of writing proposals (and coping with the rejections). The trouble with writing research proposals is that they take a great deal of time to prepare – coming up with the idea is the relatively easy part. Then a lot of time is needed to search and read the relevant literature. The preference is increasingly for bids in collaboration with other researchers and other centres. Multidisciplinary bids were encouraged, which was music to PDU ears. Almost half of one's time could easily be spent just preparing research bids. The success rate is generally low, even amongst experienced researchers. There needed to be maybe four bids a year to have any chance of regular success. The dilemma was that it appeared that a reputation was needed to be successful in bidding for research funding, and it was harder to gain a reputation for research without funding to support it.

Clinical effectiveness

In the spring of 1996 it was encouraging to learn of the appointment of a consultant to a role intended to promote 'clinical effectiveness' in the trust. The PDU Leader and Research Practitioner had some discussions with the new appointee about how best to encourage practice development and clinical effectiveness. There were values in common, with a commitment to open, democratic, decentralised decision making as a means of encouraging questioning approaches to professional practice. The teaching of critical thinking and reflective skills were agreed to be important.

The new consultant's strategy was partly about setting up or improving systems to support clinicians with information about effective clinical practice. The hope was that every ward would have quick computer access to relevant databases (such as the Cochrane database) and audit and performance data. Then, if on a ward round a question arose concerning the best way to treat whatever, the answer could be found within minutes. There were also plans for a project seeking to explore the use of information in influencing clinical decisions. Another aim was to have a multidisciplinary team to participate in a project to develop critical thinking skills. This was encouraging for the PDU, and the consultant was invited to join the PDU Steering Group, an invitation which was accepted.

Research projects

Three research projects conducted in the PDU are now described. The intention is to provide examples of how projects were set up and what they meant for participants. The first example includes a personal account by the nurse researcher concerning her involvement in a diabetes education project. The other examples are a self-medication project which was a collaboration between pharmacists and nurses, and a stroke rehabilitation project with physiotherapists and a nurse working together.

Diabetes education project

The diabetes education project illustrates in detail an example of research collaboration between the PDU and Senior Lecturer in Nursing at Leeds Metropolitan University, Mike Lowry. The personal perspective of the nurse working on the project is presented. The aim of the project was to find out what new diabetics' education needs were and involved the use of a focus group approach to find out their views of NHS support. After the focus group meeting participants were each interviewed at home by the research nurse. The nurse's account describes her experience of the project and the benefits she gained from it. The results are described more fully in Chapter 9.

Participants in the focus group were selected from patients newly referred to the hospital within the previous year and included both type I and type II diabetics. A total of eight people attended the arranged meeting. These included four diabetics, two relatives and the researchers. The nurse researcher followed up the meeting with interviews at home to explore further the issues raised in the focus group. Both the focus group meeting and the interviews were tape recorded with the consent of participants. The tapes were transcribed and content analyses were performed to identify common themes in the data. The findings of this project are presented in more detail in Chapter 9 and are to be used in discussion with service providers to examine ways of improving the service to diabetics. In addition there may be a follow up postal survey to assess the extent to which the issues identified in the focus group are relevant to a 'more representative' selection of diabetics.

The following account describes the experiences of Janis Brown, the research assistant on the project. It focuses on her thoughts and feelings about working on a research project for the first time following her successful completion of the ENB 870 post-registration research course.

My experience as a novice research assistant

Whilst I was working as a primary nurse within the PDU at Seacroft, I became involved in a research project investigating the educational needs of clients who had recently been diagnosed as suffering from diabetes mellitus. I shall briefly describe how and why I became research nurse on the project. In addition, I shall also recall the difficulties and 'highlights' of the project from a personal perspective, including how it gave opportunities for access to higher education.

Why and how I became involved

In my career of more than 20 years I have worked in a wide variety of clinical areas and I can honestly state that the education atmosphere within the PDU is exceptional, in a way that it encourages innovation and staff participation in a non-hierarchical manner. Its culture is one which encourages and motivates its staff to develop an interest in research. Research and research-based practice, as today's nurse is well aware, are essential components in planning patient care, and I was eager to learn the practical elements of nursing research. Opportunities to participate in professionally conducted research are rare and I had no experience of the research process, i.e. how a project evolves. Nevertheless, I felt confident that I would be supported by the leaders of the unit if such an opportunity arose to participate in a research project.

Clinical Forum meetings, involving staff representatives of the multidisciplinary team, occur weekly. Whilst representing the ward at the clinical forum, I learned of the planned research, which would be a 'joint venture' between Seacroft PDU and the Nursing Department of Leeds Metropolitan University. The project was to be an investigation into the educational needs of clients who were recently diagnosed as suffering from diabetes mellitus (type 1), and a volunteer was needed to assist in the research. Obviously this appeared to be the opportunity I desired to gain an insight into the process of conducting research. Those interested were asked to submit a written statement, suggesting why they should be considered for the post. Mine was accepted and I joined the research team in the New Year of 1995.

Difficulties

The initial elation and excitement of this new challenge were closely followed by doubts and anxieties concerning my ability to fulfil the role and carry out the tasks required of me. The first task was to liaise with two consultants with a special interest in diabetes. Their co-operation was needed to include patients in the project. Next there was a need to select and invite newly diagnosed diabetics and arrange with them a date for a 'focus group' meeting. Participants were encouraged to bring along a relative or friend if they wished. After attending the meeting and making notes during the session, it was my job to interview the group participants in their homes. I was also able to provide feedback and assistance to the other researchers during the transcription and analysis of the data generated from the taped interviews.

In working on the project I had several personal learning objectives. These consisted mainly of ensuring my knowledge of diabetes and its treatment was absolutely up to date. I composed an 'action learning plan' which was agreed by my ward manager. This involved spending some time in the diabetic outpatients clinic and observing the work of the diabetic nurse specialists. At the clinic I was able to experience events from the client's perspective, by 'attaching' myself to a client (who had been newly diagnosed as suffering from diabetes) for the duration of his or her first visit to the clinic. This proved to be an invaluable experience, as I gained some idea of the education clients were given at the first hospital visit (and how confusing this may appear to the client receiving this information during one visit). The issue of 'too much information at once' was identified by a client in the focus group meeting, and again during a follow-up interview. On completion of my action plan I felt satisfied that I had achieved my set goals.

Time related difficulties

During a lecture at a conference I attended in Wales a few years ago it was stated that 'in our society today, the most important and valuable thing we possess is time'. How pertinent was this observation. There were numerous barriers in preventing the research team from finding a mutually convenient time to meet to discuss the project. These included my off-duty, especially when rotated onto night duty; difficulty in contacting the lecturer at the university; one or other of us being on annual leave, or ill.

It seemed surprising that we did manage to meet at all, although when we did a great deal was achieved. One can imagine the difficulty I had negotiating a time for the focus group meeting that was mutually acceptable to all participants. Finding time to consult the notes of patients who had attended diabetic outpatients was also difficult. This was necessary to establish who had been recently diagnosed as diabetic and were suitable for the research. The criteria had to be adjusted in recognition that the majority of patients had type II diabetes.

Communication

On important issues, good communication was maintained at all times between the researchers. Some lack of communication, however, resulted in my using my own tape recorder for the interviews which I did at the participants' own homes. On one occasion the recording had picked up a lot of background noise which made transcription very difficult and time consuming.

The focus group meeting – highlight of the project

The difficulties, hard work and organisation of the project seemed worthwhile when the focus group clients and the research team met together. It would be difficult to describe the apprehension I experienced 20 minutes before the focus group was due to meet. I felt anxious wondering if the participants would remember the venue, if they would feel comfortable within the group and feel confident enough to participate and generate information. I expected that even the most experienced researcher would feel the same way before such a meeting.

The summer evening was uncomfortably warm and did nothing to cool the anxieties of the researchers. As the starting time approached one of those invited telephoned his apologies for his absence, caused by an unexpected change of his shift. This caused further apprehension. All the others arrived, much to our relief.

Fears of the researchers were needless, for it was obvious from the outset of the meeting that the diverse group (ages 40–84 years, diet, tablet and insulin controlled) were linked by the diagnosis of being 'diabetic' and had empathy and understanding of each other. The skill of the facilitator was a key contribution to its success; with minimal, skilful prompting and encouragement the group began to share experiences, anxieties and discuss the problems they had encountered as newly diagnosed diabetics. There was a great reluctance for the session to be drawn to its conclusion and it continued past its expected finishing time. A vast amount of data was generated by the group, and I was able to arrange the follow-up interviews comfortable in the knowledge that the subjects were eager to communicate their experiences and needs in relation to their diagnosis of diabetes.

Conclusion – reflecting on the experience

Obviously, I have not been able to discuss all the aspects of this project, but have touched only briefly upon the difficulties and highlights that I experienced as a novice research assistant. Throughout the project I kept a learning journal from which I have been able to reflect upon particular points of reference for further learning.

The focus group

It has been interesting to consider that at the outset of the project I had no idea of what a focus group was, how it could function, or what its role was, in terms of qualitative research. At the time, I didn't appreciate the many skills required of the facilitator who is a key person in the conduct of focus groups. On completion of the research project, I felt confident in my knowledge of focus group methodology. Now I have finished my Diploma in Practice Research and ENB 870 (for which I was granted study leave to attend), I feel I can discuss critically the focus group technique as a form of qualitative research.

The importance of the PDU philosophy

Those on the research team supported my efforts as a novice researcher by giving their expert advice, suggesting useful textbooks, and encouraging the achievement of my personal educational goals. The whole project and subsequent undertaking of the research course has been a valuable learning experience, made possible by the culture of the PDU. Patient empowerment is an important part of the PDU philosophy and this project is an example of how patients can have an influence on the service. If the project had no effect on improving the service to diabetics, it would not be worthwhile. Participants in this project said very clearly they felt valued and wanted another meeting of the group. As a result of considering the problems and opinions of these subjects, it is hoped services for the diabetic clients at Seacroft (in respect of an educational programme) will be reviewed, or further research proposed.

I believe working within the PDU has enhanced my attitude towards higher education and I hope to continue to study at Leeds Metropolitan University. In addition, I hope to be involved in future projects occurring in the PDU.

The self-medication research project

The first major success was in getting funds to support a patient self-medication project. This was a one year study which aimed to test if patients going through a structured self-medication programme did better on knowledge and compliance outcomes than a similar group going through the usual preparation. The grant paid for a nurse to work part time on the project with a pharmacist. The research involved interviewing patients in hospital with follow-up visits to patients after discharge. The nurse involved, Liz Hayward, had just completed the ENB 870 research course and was keen to apply her newly acquired skills. The pharmacist was embarking on her own postgraduate research for her PhD. The project was a great success, with a very positive endorsement for the self-medication programme over the usual approach of 'can I just tell you about your medicines before you go home?' There were publications in the *British Medical Journal*, a presentation at the Geriatric Society Conference and even an interview of the pharmacist Cathy Lowe by the Radio 4 'Medicine Now' programme. This was just what was needed for the PDU – a national profile and recognition of the value of research carried out by clinical staff.

However, there was a major lesson to be learnt from this project. It was one thing to prove that a particular approach was worthwhile and good for patients. It was entirely another to put it into practice. Three years after the research was completed resources were still not available to support the full implementation of the self-medication programme on all of the wards. The issue was the pharmacy technician time needed to fill and label the individual medicine bottles required for the programme. It was possible to support just a few patients at any one time on self-medication, but the constraint on implementation was very frustrating and demoralising for those involved. Efforts to secure funding continue. Tenacity is a virtue.

Pharmacist Cathy Lowe's account

Background

I took up post on the PDU at its inception in December 1991. The ethos of the PDU has already been outlined in previous chapters, that is, multidisciplinary working, encouraging research and development of professional practice. When I came into post one of my main objectives was to investigate the feasibility of setting up a self-medication programme on the unit. The concept of self-medication fitted in with the philosophy of the PDU in a number of ways. Firstly, it needed the participation of different professions. Secondly, it empowered patients through giving them informed choice and thus working in partnership with them. I had previous experience of working in both medicine and psychiatry for the elderly and knew the difficulties that these patients could often have with their medication. The problem is often one of a lack of compliance with medication after discharge from hospital. I had also reviewed the literature and was aware of the scale of the problem with its effect on patient morbidity and the subsequent cost of this. The difficulty facing health care workers is knowing what can be done to improve the situation. The literature search had shown that there was no single intervention that increased compliance in the long term but rather a combination of strategies. The strength of a self-medication programme is that it combines a number of strategies that are known to improve compliance, that is, medication review and rationalisation, assessment of patient needs and education. However, there has been little objective evaluation of such a mix of approaches on compliance. In these days of evidence-based practice we felt that there was a need to have proof of the value of a programme before we used it. So the idea of undertaking a piece of research was born.

Developing the study

Once we had decided to undertake the research project we had to focus our ideas and write a protocol. It became increasingly clear that we would need to find funding if the work was to be of any quality. At the same time Yorkshire Regional Health Authority invited candidates to apply for research monies. We successfully applied for this money and received sufficient to employ a nurse for three days a week to work with me on the project. The funding for this lasted for 14 months. A working group was formed consisting of nurses and pharmacists to oversee the work which Liz Hayward (the research nurse) and I were to undertake. In the early days we did not have a doctor because two of the three consultants had not been appointed and the posts were filled by locums. The medical director gave us his wholehearted support but commitments did not allow him to become actively involved. A consultant also joined us once the study had begun.

When designing the self-medication programme we first assessed the type of patients we were likely to have. The then four wards were 'medicine for the elderly' and so we felt that an intensive programme which had three levels of supervision with a detailed initial assessment would be appropriate. The design of the protocol was critical and we drew on a lot of in-house expertise. The research advisory group was a vital source of advice for methodology.

The self-medication study outline

The study was a randomised controlled trial. The process of selecting a ward for admission of patients was random, so the study group was on one ward and the control group on another.

The study group

After referral of a patient by the primary nurse to the pharmacist both assessed the patient using a structured assessment form covering the patient's understanding of their medication, their ability to read labels and their ability to cope with closures (bottles, packaging, etc.). The pharmacist explained the medication to the patient and summarised the explanation on a drug reminder chart. The self-medication programme had three stages of increasing independence.

- At stage 1 the nurse handed the patient a box containing their intended medicines. The patient was supervised taking the medication and the nurse intervened only when necessary if the patient was about to make a mistake.
- Stage 2 was the same as for stage 1, except that the patient was expected to request their medication at the appropriate time: 30 minutes was allowed to elapse before the nurse reminded the patient.
- At stage 3 the patient had total responsibility for taking their medication, which was stored in a locker beside their bed. A nurse performed a daily tablet count.

The control group

All patients received their medicines on drug rounds, and were given brief explanations of their medications on discharge.

On discharge, patients were sent home with two weeks, supply of medication. Patients in both study and control groups received written information listing drugs and dosage. They received a visit from the research nurse at 10 days after discharge and were interviewed using a structured questionnaire. A tablet count was performed. Repeat interviews and tablet counts were conducted at three months.

Practical aspects of the study

Once the protocol was designed the research nurse and I had the task of implementing it. This proved to be no small undertaking!

The study was introduced to the PDU one ward at a time. A combination of staff meetings and one-to-one tuition was used to explain what staff needed to do. Each ward had a copy of the study protocol. I visited the wards every day and carried a bleep and so was always on hand to sort out any problems. The research nurse Liz also visited the wards on each of her three days a week on the project. We found that old patterns of work die hard and it took a lot of effort on all sides to change this. One problem occurred when drug charts were sent to pharmacy for the discharge medication to be prepared. Pharmacy did not know which patients were included in the study and so did not dispense the medication appropriately. This involved a lot of duplicated work on the part of pharmacy. Difficulties also arose if the doctor changed the drug regime of a self-medicating patient and did not tell the patient or nursing staff. Other problems occurred with the process of referral to the self-medication programme. This was erratic and in the end Liz and I scrutinised all patients ourselves.

How did the PDU help?

The culture on the PDU helped in a number of ways. The most important factor for me was that research was a fundamental expectation of the unit rather than something I had to fight to do. In previous posts (two at teaching hospitals) much was talked of doing research but when it came to actually doing it there were always blocks. Firstly there was a considerable hierarchy to ascend when you had an idea. Secondly, there had to be agreement between various groups. Thirdly, if you got that far before exhaustion or cynicism set in, the original idea would be killed by pressure of time. The PDU had a number of advantages in that there was a flat management structure with a prevailing culture which allowed anyone to have an idea regardless of the position held within the organisation. These ideas were actively sought and listened to. Wherever possible the individual was encouraged to pursue an idea and was given as much practical support as possible. My manager recognised that research was not a closet activity and allowed me time to pursue the study at the expense of other objectives.

The study had the total support of the medical director and the manager of the department. This proved vital not only for the encouragement and affirmation they gave, but also for the economic muscle power when funding was necessary.

Networking and publication

The study has been presented to a number of conferences, including the British Geriatric Society. It was published in the *British Medical*

Journal, which has resulted in letters from all over the UK and indeed the world. The work was also discussed when I was invited to be interviewed on Radio 4's 'Medicine Now' programme.

Theory into practice

I would like to be able to report that since the study finished in 1993 we have had a fully operational self-medication programme on all wards on the PDU. Sadly this is not the case for one very crucial reason – money! There is a time commitment to self-medication for both nurses and pharmacy staff. For nurses the extra time involved in the early stages of the programme is offset by the decrease in time when patients are fully independent. Unfortunately the same cannot be said for pharmacy. There is a fairly major time commitment from both pharmacist and the technical staff in the dispensing. This costs extra, and when this was calculated the hospital management were unwilling to fund it. Since that time there has been some fairly heavy lobbying from nurses, pharmacists and doctors to no avail.

The stroke physiotherapy pilot project

Another success was to get a small research grant to fund a small pilot physiotherapy project. It was thought that if larger bids were unsuccessful then perhaps it would work if bids for amounts under £1000 to fund pilot work might get us established on the ladder. The pilot work would help us build up our expertise and experience, and might help a larger bid later on the basis of the pilot work. This project involved physiotherapists in research for the first time in the PDU and was jointly led by the research practitioner and senior physiotherapist. Other physiotherapists were involved from time to time gathering data, thus broadening opportunities for promoting a questioning culture. There was a delay of three months initially because of a misunderstanding about the process for transferring the research grant from region to the hospital. Once this was resolved the work got under way.

The project itself was concerned with trying to measure functional ability in people with stroke before and after weekends. At Seacroft and in most other hospitals, physiotherapy for stroke patients is only provided on weekdays. Anecdotal evidence suggested that there may be a decline in functional ability after a weekend 'resting' without physiotherapy. However, measuring day-to-day changes in functional ability is difficult, since any changes are actually quite subtle. Using a technique called TELER (Le Roux, 1993), physiotherapists and the PDU research practitioner measured stroke patients' function for a range of abilities related to movement and mobility.

As an exercise in involving staff who had not worked on research before, the project was successful. Part of the grant paid for training in using the TELER technique. Some difficulties arose when opportunities for measurement were missed. This was understandable given the problems with physiotherapy staffing levels, and the fact that some were on a rotation between two sites, which meant training new staff each time the changeover occurred. Data recording improved when monthly feedback sessions were organised. There were sometimes difficulties in recruiting patients to the study, partly because the admission rate for people with stroke dropped as soon as the study started, and also because workload pressures meant patient treatment took priority. This did not create any major problems except to delay the progress of the project.

Whilst this project was successful in involving physiotherapy staff in research, this put considerable pressure on them in addition to their already heavy workload. The PDU multidisciplinary philosophy placed great pressures on therapy staff in general because of their relatively small numbers compared with nurses. As well as research, they contributed much to audit activity and various other aspects of PDU work, and it is to their credit that they were able to manage it all.

The findings of the project indicated that for the stroke patients included in the pilot, most maintained levels of functional activity over weekends rather than showing improvements or a decline. The conclusion of the project was delayed by three months when the research practitioner was required to work full time on a ward to cover for nursing staff shortages. Whilst this was useful in other ways such as the identification of areas for future research, it did little to show that management was fully committed to supporting research activity.

Conclusion

The PDU has been successful in enabling research to be done in practice settings and involving staff from a range of disciplines for the first time in research. Through the research advisory group the PDU has forged links with higher education and has been able to tap into expertise not previously available. It has also successfully demonstrated how it is possible for clinically based staff to collaborate with researchers in universities on research. Universities are very keen to do research as their income partly depends on it. They also need access to clinical settings for both the placement of their students and for research. There is mutual benefit in working together on research as a means of closing the theory–practice gap, demystifying research and motivating staff to explore their practice more rigorously and find ways of providing a better service to patients. However, generally speaking, some managers do not see research as a priority and much work is still required to persuade them otherwise.

Chapter 8
Staff empowerment

Sally Casley

The **PDU model** is underpinned by a distinct philosophy of practice and characterised by six essential elements, each of which is explored in detail in this part of the book. It was recognised at the outset, however, that the essential foundation for all of the other elements was the empowerment of the individuals working within the unit.

Key aspirations, therefore, when establishing the PDU were to create an environment where:

- individuals at all levels and in all disciplines could become actively involved in developments on the unit and would feel safe in doing so
- decision making would be moved closer to the patient, so that staff from all disciplines delivering care would be making most of the day-to-day decisions
- opportunities were created within the workplace for development of staff at all levels, in order to enable them to build the skills and knowledge needed to take part in the venture.

The empowerment of staff is such a fundamental part of the PDU's approach that to some extent many of the issues have already been discussed in detail in earlier chapters. The purpose of this chapter, therefore, is not to repeat this material, which amply sets out the unit's beliefs about empowerment and the frameworks established to develop and support this in a multidisciplinary context. Rather, it is to illustrate some of the benefits of this empowerment by reference

153

first to the development of primary nursing within the unit and later through the words of some of the members of the PDU team themselves. To start, however, we will begin by considering some of the developments in leadership of the PDU and their influence on the empowerment of staff.

Leadership and empowerment in the PDU

Staff moving from St George's to Seacroft Hospital were anxious about caring for acute medical patients as well as the longer stay medical patients they had been used to caring for. They were comfortable with working closely as a multidisciplinary team but needed to be able to transpose this multidisciplinary model in their new setting whilst acquiring new skills to care for acutely ill patients. To enable staff to be able to make this transition in practice they needed support mechanisms so that they could grow in their new role and feel empowered to make these decisions from a knowledge base.

Traditionally medical staff have led the ward teams with nurses and professions allied to medicine falling into line. The philosophy of the PDU is to value the contributions of all members of staff of the multidisciplinary team in promoting high quality care and practice development. Staff needed to be encouraged to question all aspects of practice and recognise that there is a need to accept well considered risk taking as part of development.

As this was breaking away from previous hospital working ethos, the Clinical Director, Hospital Services Manager and PDU Leader had a key role to play if this questioning culture was to evolve in the newly merged hospital environment. They wanted to enable staff to grow professionally. By giving staff autonomy they would empower staff to make decisions.

The Clinical Director, Hospital Services Manager and PDU Leader needed to motivate staff to make the move from St George's to Seacroft a positive change. Initially their leadership style was to have a strong visible presence so that they were accessible and available to support staff on a daily basis. They are still remembered for their energy and enthusiasm. The first Clinical Leader of the PDU has been described by one member of staff as 'all encompassing'. Once she started a project whether staff initially felt it was a good idea or not they would be swept along by her 'overwhelming enthusiasm'. Staff talk about how they were made to feel valued as an equal member of the team which gave them the confidence to question both their own and others' practice. This had a snowball effect and was enhanced by a number of projects undertaken by staff of all grades.

Leaders needed to be visible and approachable if the organisation was to evolve as a multidisciplinary organisation. 'An effective leader knows that the ultimate task of leadership is to create human energies and human vision' (Mullins, 1989) . This view of leadership encompasses what the leaders of the PDU have always tried to achieve. A change in both managerial leadership and clinical leadership has not changed this philosophy.

When the second PDU Leader came into post he made a conscious decision to change the leadership style in order to raise the academic awareness of the work of the PDU.

Networking and dissemination were also seen as positive ways of enhancing the work on the PDU and another way of empowering staff. He started evaluating the work completed so far and looked at ways of enhancing academic rigour. The role of the Quality Assurance Nurse who had previously supported the first PDU Leader was changed to become that of Research Practitioner. Much of the work carried out by the Quality Assurance Nurse had been related to local research and audit. The change in title and job description gave clarity to his role and brought with it a sharper focus on development of specific research interests within the unit. It also removed the title of nurse, which meant that it formally became a role to support all disciplines, rather than just the nursing staff as the previous title may have suggested.

In November 1993 a visit to Lille in France was arranged in order to compare and contrast both nursing and management styles. This visit had a high profile and, as well as being of educational benefit, it also sent a message to staff that they were being encouraged to think of national and international contacts and contrasts. The need to provide value for money was another reason for the visit and gave the managers an opportunity to see how alternative systems worked in practice. The foci for the development of excellence in Lille were care and clinical excellence, training and education, research and service development. The visit demonstrated to the PDU how interlinked clinical and management services were. It demonstrated a need to review further education for the ward manager based on management and budget training which was the model used by the Lille hospitals.

The Clinical Director through management consultancy work had talked to Mike Pedler (a management consultant) about how the

PDU had been conceived and the model used to bring two hospitals together. As a result of this contact, at a later stage the work of the PDU was filmed and featured in a BBC management educational video called 'The Learning Organisation'. This again reinforced to staff the confidence of the management in the work of the PDU where staff delivering care were also initiating developments to help shape the health service for the people in Leeds.

Prior to April 1996 the PDU goals were always part of the hospital business plan. In order to develop these goals multidisciplinary 'time-out' days were planned for the Medical Directorate before it became part of a large Division of Medicine with a different organisational structure.

The 'time-out' days would be used to write the management and clinical agenda so that all disciplines were able to contribute towards the yearly plan. The PDU Leader was responsible for documenting the clinical objectives and disseminating this information in the medical Directorate. The progress of the plan would then be reviewed on a regular basis with the Hospital Services Manager, Clinical Director (Senior Medical Consultant), Therapy Services Manager and PDU Leader. Individual members of staff would be supported to complete their work throughout the year thus empowering staff further.

Empowerment in action

To feel the benefits of empowerment, staff needed to experience how this would change their daily practice. Within the unit it became an expectation that staff would want to be included in projects (part of the concept of 'norms for excellence' from West (1990) discussed in earlier chapters), which was reinforced through the daily work of the unit. Staff responded positively to this expectation, which was backed also by practical support for work undertaken. As they were choosing an area of personal interest which they felt would improve the quality of patient care, individuals also became able to see the process of change from start to finish.

Individuals working within the unit were therefore more likely to ask themselves why they were carrying out a particular activity and its relevance to the individual patient. They also experienced how to implement a change in practice and the different barriers which might stop change taking place.

Within the unit, individuals at a number of levels and from different disciplines have been able to initiate projects which have resulted in changes in practice. Not all projects have been completed successfully of course – some because of the impact of organisational changes and others for a variety of reasons including change in personnel and lack of resources, including time and money. In itself this is not serious and is a natural phenomenon where innovation is attempted and planned risk taking is encouraged. It only becomes problematic where this outcome becomes the norm and damages the belief within the team that they can bring about change and will be taken seriously by others.

Primary nursing and staff empowerment

Primary nursing was seen as a key way of empowering the nursing staff. The first PDU Leader initiated a retrospective study to see if this was the case. The project team focused on three areas: interdisciplinary and ward communication, primary nursing and job satisfaction, and patients views about primary nursing. The project team consisted of primary nurses, a Senior Nurse and the PDU Leader.

Primary nursing was established on all the wards within the Department of Medicine rather than just the PDU. The length of time primary nursing had been established and the implementation of the model varied from ward to ward, as this had been taken forward by individual ward teams rather than as a single top-down exercise.

The nursing team had expressed the view that although nurses generally said that primary nursing was better for patients and there was a wealth of published information describing how to implement it, there was still little available published data on evaluation and proven benefits to staff and patients following its implementation. The project team wanted to evaluate the effectiveness within their own department by evaluating the three areas detailed above.

To evaluate interdisciplinary and ward communication a survey was designed for use with professions other than nursing to establish:

- their knowledge of how primary nursing worked in practice
- how easy it was to identify which primary nurse was responsible for individual patients
- the effectiveness of ward communication prior to and following the introduction of primary nursing
- how integrated multidisciplinary patient records were prior to and following the introduction of primary nursing
- any change in the quality of information received about individual patients since the introduction of primary nursing
- the overall opinion of its value or disadvantages.

The conclusions drawn from this questionnaire were that the majority of the professionals felt that primary nursing was a change for the better and improved care but that more work was needed on effective channels of communication and coordination when the primary nurse was absent.

Recommendations which followed included ensuring that all wards used an information board with the name and/or photograph of the primary nurses and that there was an improvement of the quality of the patient assessment document and care plans, firstly by holding monthly peer audit of nursing and multidisciplinary care plans and secondly by enabling all sisters to attend a study day on 'Keeping the Record Straight' in order to raise awareness of legal implications of poor documentation and the law with regard to record keeping by health care professionals.

The second part of the project asked about primary nursing and job satisfaction. The project team decided that rather than frame the questions around their own experiences and assumptions they would send an open questionnaire.

The results of this survey appeared to demonstrate that primary nursing and job satisfaction were linked as the nursing staff saw primary nursing as a way of devolving power to trained nurses which put them in a position where they were accountable and autonomous in the delivery of care. The study revealed, however, that nurses do not automatically gain job satisfaction by taking on the role of primary nurse. The role needs continuous support and evaluation to empower nurses to fulfil the role effectively and gain job satisfaction.

Recommendations included clearly written information on every ward about role definitions within the ward team with an emphasis being placed on the responsibilities of the primary nurse for prescribing care, a team building strategy for each ward with the focus on the F-grade sister who was to become the ward's clinical leader, regular meetings for primary nurses, an induction course for associate nurses who wish to become primary nurses and the appointment of a deputy primary nurse who can deputise for the primary nurse when the primary nurse is on leave.

The third part of the study was to look at the patients' views of primary nursing, which were again ascertained by the use of a questionnaire. The results of this survey revealed that patients expressed themselves highly satisfied that their needs had been met by nursing staff. The majority of patients had been given an explanation of what primary nursing was and had had daily contact with their primary nurse. Recommendations from this survey were that all patients should receive an explanation about primary nursing and that information at the patient's bedside should be available to assist in this process. Primary nurses or their deputy should discuss the patient's care and treatment at least once a day with the other members of their primary team and patients should be actively involved in their care with open and free access to their care plan. As a result of this project the recommendations were taken forward through a number of multidisciplinary project groups, as well as being fed into discussions with the hospital managers, in order to influence wider hospital practice.

After the completion of the primary nursing evaluation project, a ward sister development programme was established as a hospital-wide initiative for all ward sisters, reflecting the growing view of them as having key roles in the empowerment of their ward teams in the delivery of patient care. This programme was workshop-based initially, with time out days away from the clinical area. With the programme being implemented across the hospital rather than just within the PDU, the unit and its work on primary nursing were seen to have exerted a significant influence on the development and the PDU Leader was responsible for leading and coordinating these workshops with the support of the Head of Professional Development.

Topics for both the workshops for the ward manager and clinical sister revolved around role clarification. There had been a conscious decision to move away from the title of ward sister to ward manager when the ward budgets were devolved. This meant the ward manager needed to acquire management skills in order to manage the ward budget effectively. The role of the F-grade sister was developed into that of clinical leader for the ward supporting the primary nurses and coordinating clinical developments on their own wards.

Multidisciplinary documentation

Other work arising from the focus on primary nursing and the recommendations from the survey was related to the issue of record keeping. A multidisciplinary project group was set up at an early stage in the PDU's development, in order to develop communication between the different members of the team. This work has been described in detail in Chapter 6. Later work built on the original documents created by this project group in order to further refine the system. The PDU Leader and Research Practitioner coordinated this work which meant meeting with a team representing each discipline to decide what core information was needed on the assessment document. Each discipline then discussed this with colleagues from the same profession before further discussions took place within the project team. The work of this team took 18 months to complete as a result of the extensive multidisciplinary discussions both across the hospital and involving the community services. The printed versions of the multidisciplinary assessment booklet and the admissions sheet were subsequently implemented across the Department of Medicine. The key characteristic of these documents was that (although as with most documents it is rare to find anyone who was happy with all aspects of them) they were truly designed by the people who would be using them, and were therefore more likely to meet the needs of everyday practice.

In addition to the work on multidisciplinary records, the PDU Leader worked with one of the hospital's Clinical Nurse Specialists who had a personal interest in raising the profile of documentation. Using the 'Just for the Record' training folder produced by the NHS Management Executive, workshops were run for primary nurses and others to attend. Each ward was issued with a copy of the folder. Before and after the workshops, ward documentation was audited by practitioners themselves and results of the audit demonstrated that the workshops had been beneficial as there was an improvement in the clarity of clinical documentation.

The work carried out in these workshops was seen as a way of empowering staff to give a quality service, by helping them to reflect on their own everyday practice and its importance to the quality of the patient's care, and by building in, as an intrinsic part of the programme, opportunities for practitioners to audit practice within their own wards and to initiate appropriate changes in practice. At the same time the work also mirrored the national concerns about nursing documentation and the need to write accurate and timely information. The work of the PDU was enhancing the national strategy for nurses as dictated by the UK Central Council.

Overall, the development of primary nursing was a useful vehicle for the development of empowerment in a number of ways. In addition to its effects on the primary nurses themselves, it also had a positive impact on other roles within the ward team, from complementing the development of the sisters' roles, to the creation and support of new, developmental roles within the ward team for associate nurses and for the health care support workers. Within the multidisciplinary team, it provided an effective focal point for communication and stimulated detailed work on interdis-

ciplinary communication which led to the development of the
unit's multidisciplinary records system and other related developments.

The primary nursing system on each ward was rarely perfect and
indeed created its own problems at times, but what it did achieve was
the creation of a framework at the level of the ward which supported
the PDU objective of empowering of staff at all levels and involving
them in a broad range of debates and project work related to the
care of their patients.

Personal perspectives

A cross-section of the multidisciplinary team were asked if they felt
working in a PDU empowered them in their daily practice. Their
comments reflect the clinical staff's views of day-to-day experiences.

A consultant's comments

As a consultant physician with an interest in the elderly, I consider
that effective multidisciplinary team work is central to good patient
care. The PDU provides an environment which supports current
good practice while encouraging a questioning and innovative
approach leading to improvements in practice. The philosophy of
current practice supporting innovation and development, which
then feeds back into improved practice, is central to the success of
the unit. This is encouraged in a number of ways:

- a willingness among all staff, particularly those in senior positions
  such as consultants and ward managers, to discuss and support
  new ideas and approaches
- posts within the unit with a development role, enabling staff to
  discuss new ideas (e.g. PDU Clinical Leader and a Clinical Nurse
  Specialist) and fostering links with other bodies such as the
  College of Health and local universities
- arenas for presentation, discussion and dissemination of new
  developments such as the Clinical Forum, the Research Advisory
  Group and multidisciplinary Clinical Audit sessions.

From a personal perspective, working in the PDU has a number
of direct benefits:

- working as part of a positive and enthusiastic team with a strong
  commitment to patient care

- frequent meetings and discussions with staff from all disciplines about ideas, projects and developments to improve care
- a willingness of staff to take part in formal research projects.

These make the PDU a stimulating, challenging and rewarding place to work.

A ward manager

I have recently started work within the PDU at Seacroft Hospital, having had a conventional background of general nursing prior to this where research, although seen as important, was regarded very much as secondary and not as an integral part of the nursing process' and decision making and new ideas came almost always from the most senior members of the ward. My prior knowledge of what a PDU meant in real terms was therefore very limited. However I did have strong views that all members of the ward team have a valuable contribution to make in order to continually strive to improve patient care.

With this in mind I took up my new post and was at once struck by how well the ward worked as a team. This included not only the nursing staff but medical, nursing, domestic, and all professions allied to medicine. Most importantly the patients were included in this team.

All the individual members of staff had a clear idea of the important role they played in providing good patient care and therefore very much felt valued as individuals.

They seemed to have built a trust and understanding between the team whereby they felt able to express their ideas to each other. This does not mean there were not the usual disputes that occur in every working environment, but on the whole, with guidance the team were able to work through these areas of disagreement and thereby strengthened the team further.

I was surprised to find myself feeling slightly uncomfortable and maybe even threatened by this staff and patient empowerment as I had been much more used to a hierarchical method of care delivery.

I am pleased to say that although in theory I always believed in allowing every member of the ward a voice in the running of the ward, I can now fully appreciate the benefits of doing so. I very much see part of my role now as continuing to allow all members of the team a voice in the care delivery on the ward and thereby empowering each and every one of them to have a say in the daily running of the ward whilst continuing to show them that they are all valued as people.

A ward manager who moved from a PDU ward to a non-PDU ward

While working as a ward manager on the PDU I learnt the importance of starting change from the bottom upwards and that regardless of grade, everyone has the right to question. I strongly believe that the ward team does not just relate to the immediate ward team but encompasses physiotherapists, occupational therapists, the dietitians and all other professionals allied to medicine who have contact with the patients. The important factor is we all work together.

Working on the PDU, on reflection, empowers you because you can challenge care and, because staff working in the same area have the same philosophy, they do not feel threatened by being questioned about their practice. All staff are encouraged to take control by initiating care. This in time filters through and all staff feel able to challenge one another.

The PDU was about changing traditions on the ward. Before the development of the PDU the sister or charge nurse used to take sole charge of the ward round and case conference without other members of the nursing staff. With the introduction of primary nursing this was no longer the case. Obviously this did not come easily to everyone but, with support, staff slowly realised that they cared for the patients day in, day out, so it made sense that they discussed the patient with the medical staff including the consultant and with other members of the multidisciplinary team. Staff were encouraged to question care and why they had decided to act in a certain way. As a result I felt my ward was homely and that staff pulled together. They knew what being a team meant. There were no grievances or gossip. The ward atmosphere was pleasant and cheerful. Staff shared in ideas as to how patients should be cared for in order to maximise patient independence. An example of this would be the physiotherapist looking with nursing staff how to handle a patient.

This meant staff needed to be able to give their best to understand what were trying to achieve whether this related to diagnosis or any aspect of care delivery. For staff to be able to give their best they need appropriate training which was seen as part of the PDU philosophy.

Moving to a non-PDU ward I found the atmosphere very different. It was very nurse and doctor orientated. By this I mean that the ward did not have the same team spirit. On the PDU ward I would ask the nursing staff if they would explain to me why they had put bed rails on a patient's bed or why they had catheterised a patient and I would be given an explanation. If I ask the same questions now, staff feel they are being criticised and become defensive. The major difference is that staff react rather than initiate in their day-to-day activities. Staff wait to be told to refer to the physiotherapist or occupational therapist. There appears to be no sense of multidisciplinary working or understanding that closely working together and sharing practice will be of benefit to the patient.

Unfortunately not all the projects started by the PDU have been completed, because of the time it takes to get a project off the ground. Some other projects were not rolled out so the benefits were not felt by all the wards.

I feel it was the philosophies of the people who originally set up the PDU who helped empower me in my role as a ward manager. I think I would still feel empowered by my experiences on the PDU if the PDU did not exist in the future.

A ward manager comparing a PDU and a non-PDU ward

The three most significant differences between the PDU ward and non-PDU ward were the involvement of the multidisciplinary team which I attributed to the different needs of the patients (I had previously worked on a Reception Unit for acutely ill medical patients), the involvement of all grades of staff from the multidisciplinary team in decision making and meetings to plan patient care, and members of staff asking me for my opinion which they valued and acted upon.

As a ward manager for a PDU ward I feel more time is needed to undertake the role so that I can achieve the expectations of me to fulfil my practice development role, management role and clinical role. Due to time limitations clinical issues usually take priority.

Support from senior management has been limited due to our trust merging which has meant senior managers have been involved in reorganisation. My main support has been from my peers and Personnel Department.

It is difficult to isolate the difference between a PDU ward and a non-PDU ward as I am not able to compare one ward with another ward. In general terms I found the non-PDU area to be more self-sufficient, not looking outside their own working environment to solve problems because of their specialism. There was no multidisciplinary team working, which in retrospect would have been useful.

When I took the post as a ward manager on the PDU I thought I understood what the PDU was trying to achieve but on reflection I feel I needed more preparation to be able to fulfil the practice development role. It has become another ball to juggle which needs time.

A staff nurse who 'acted up' on a PDU ward

I acted up on a PDU ward to cover a period of maternity leave. I was already working on a PDU ward so my main objective was to 'test the water' and discover, without prior commitment to a permanent contract, if the role would be appropriate for my needs.

I was not concerned about support in my new role as I knew the organisation well and was secure in the knowledge that I could phone a number of people irrespective of the time if I needed support or advice. Everyone I approached always had time to discuss any issue ranging from trivial items to more complex issues.

I felt the level of responsibility was reasonable, challenging and quite exciting. The new skills I acquired in the secondment were a broader view of the hospital instead of being blinkered by my own vision, the opportunity to enhance my existing knowledge and increase my confidence. I now feel confident when working with senior managers.

The secondment was a good move for training purposes. When I reverted to being an E-grade staff nurse after the secondment, I felt restless. Following feedback from managers, my increased personal confidence enabled me to apply successfully for a permanent F-grade sister post.

An occupational therapist

At Seacroft Hospital the PDU began working towards its accreditation in 1991–2 as the elderly care wards at St George's Hospital were transferred to Seacroft to integrate into one unit with the general medical wards.

The occupational therapy staff were transferred across to the new unit at the same level which meant one part time therapist and a full time assistant to each pair of wards.

Occupational therapy staff were involved with the development of the PDU concept. The keenness of the project leaders to have multidisciplinary involvement necessitated the attendance of occupational therapists at as many meetings as possible related to different innovations. The occupational therapists had to select which meetings they could attend and it became necessary to involve the occupational therapy assistants in some of the project groups reporting back to the qualified staff. This has led to more involvement and satisfaction for all levels of staff.

The weekly Clinical Forum is where we got feedback about different projects and where we could discuss the implications for occupational therapy of any of the new initiatives. It also provided a means for us to update other members of the team on new developments in our own area.

On the PDU the multidisciplinary team worked well. Nursing staff and other disciplines were very aware of what the occupational therapy services had to offer, and where the occupational therapy role fitted into the team. A benefit of this team working was that referrals came early which reflected the planning ability of the nursing staff.

Occupational therapists and assistants working closely on the wards felt valued as part of the ward team and their knowledge and help was often sought after by other disciplines on the unit.

Discharge planning seemed less of a problem on the PDU where the multidisciplinary team worked well together with early recognition of problems aided by weekly case conferences and meetings.

Occupational therapists working on the PDU felt that staff on the unit were aware of what services could be offered and how the social details of the patients' care were often needed in communication with the occupational therapy staff to help with the discharge arrangements.

The occupational therapists felt that they got greater job satisfaction from working with an astute team. Nursing students were often directed towards the occupational therapy service by their supervisors as the nursing staff were aware that the occupational therapy input was an essential part of the patients' rehabilitation and discharge arrangements.

The slightly above average levels of occupational therapy staff in the unit helped us to respond successfully to requests for input, and helped to ensure successful team work and cooperation with all concerned to deliver quality care for our patients.

A health care assistant

I have worked on the PDU for three years. When I was offered the position I did not understand what the unit was or its function within the hospital. During the time that I have worked there, my understanding has become much clearer.

I feel it a privilege to work as a health care assistant on such a unit as you are encouraged to develop any skills and potential you have. I have been supported to attend various courses. I have already completed the BTEC Level One and Level Two course and am now attending the BTEC Health and Science Studies course which will give me the qualification to go on and do my nurse training which is what I hope to do. Since starting the courses my job with the ward has changed. I have become more involved with different aspects of nursing.

On the PDU each member of staff is treated alike. Everyone has valid points and opinions which are listened to and taken on board. An example of this is that a few months ago a colleague (who is also a health care assistant) and I, along with other members of the multi-disciplinary team, were asked to make a presentation to the Trust Directors. Doctors, ward sisters and hospital managers were also present to hear us. The talk was about the unit and our roles within it. It was the longest and most nerve-wracking time of my life but afterwards I was told that my colleague and I were the first two health care assistants to be part of such a talk to management. After doing this I felt very excited and also honoured that we were encouraged to speak about our roles. I felt that this shows how things are changing within the nursing profession.

The PDU is a very interesting place to work, in that we are able to see different ideas put into practice, meeting visitors from many different places as far away as France and, knowing that we are all part of it in some way.

The unit has got such a lot to offer but it is up to the individual to use the resources available. It plays a very important part within the hospital setting and deserves all the credit it can get. Everyone should be aware of what the PDU is and what its functions are.

Times are definitely changing within the health professions and it is up to everyone to make sure those changes are positive and that the patient is the one to benefit most. This is what the PDU is striving to do but it takes everyone to contribute in some way or another to help achieve a positive outcome.

A staff nurse involved in making a change in clinical practice

Implementing a no-lifting policy was one of the early projects embarked upon by the PDU. I had chosen to come and work on the PDU because of its philosophy and a wish to develop personally and professionally. I also had a personal interest in a no-lifting policy as I had previously sustained a back injury. When I came for my interview for the post on the PDU I was told I wouldn't be expected to lift as I would be asked to implement the no-lifting policy. I felt that I had full responsibility to work within budget but was given the autonomy to choose the necessary equipment and to select the appropriate methods of implementation.

Although it was flattering to receive the responsibility and the freedom to work autonomously, I did feel isolated on occasions. I felt at times managers were asking when the policy was ready for implementation and not what they could do to help.

I did receive a great deal of support from the senior physiotherapist, but her own workload inhibited her practical help with training in the early stages. Working together was of benefit in order to present a united front especially as the physiotherapist already knew the staff. The PDU Leader was also approachable and supportive.

As I was new to the PDU I would have found additional support helpful. I would have like to have arranged meetings with managers at the beginning and also have identified which staff on the PDU already had an interest in a no-lifting policy.

Making change is a lengthy process, although easier that I had anticipated. Factors which helped to implement the changes were commitment to the policy myself, support from senior staff members in particular the senior physiotherapist, and that staff knew the project was supported by senior managers.

Factors that hindered the change were a lack of consistency in the way the ward was managed, time to train all staff on their practical techniques and some negative and resistant attitudes of staff to change.

Whilst instituting this change I felt I had sufficient knowledge about the subject and that in taking this responsibility I was developing personally from the experience. I saw this as advantageous for gaining promotion. I would have liked more knowledge about change management at which I have looked more closely since completing the project. I have discovered management processes and methods I could have used. I felt a great sense of achievement when the policy was implemented.

If I was asked to do it again I would liaise more closely with the medical staff in order to reduce the risk of any confusion in an emergency situation. I feel that most of the problems I encountered in implementing the policy were due to the fact that I was new to the unit.

A physiotherapist's view on implementing a policy for safer moving and handling

My responsibilities mainly revolved around teaching specific techniques with various pieces of equipment and assessing those trained by me for competence and safety. I probably was not prepared for just how much work was involved and would be in future, in planning ahead for training sessions and problem-solving sessions. I learnt a lot during the time and feel that the most important single issue is getting staff to own something. If you can do this, the rest is a piece of cake!

Barriers to implementing the change were that there was never enough time to do everything we wanted to do. At times staff morale was low which also caused difficulties when we had a number of particularly heavy patients without enough of the specific equipment we needed in place. There were also particular difficulties with educating staff at weekends which posed particular problems for both staff and patients because there were two different approaches to handling them. The most difficult barrier to overcome was staff attitudes. Most staff were interested but did not always see the need to change their practice which appeared to have worked for years.

On reflection, I know now how to advertise changes in a better way. We have prepared to 'roll out' the no-lifting policy on to other wards so I have paved the way by providing photographs of the equipment and the handling techniques as well as posters and practical interactions in the techniques necessary to avoid lifting. I have also asked ward managers for time at their individual ward meetings to discuss the way forward and encourage ownership of the project by the ward staff.

There was a particular point in time when I realised that not only were staff asking for help and advice, but they were using the equipment purchased for the project in a confident and experienced manner. I also had two supportive physiotherapy assistants who were able to reinforce the advice already given.

A hospital manager's view of practice development

The research and development of practice involving every discipline is essential. We can no longer ignore the need to break down the perceived barriers between clinical professions and 'the management' and between the different clinical professions. The objective now is no longer just to talk about achieving better patient care by greater working together, but to be seen to do it.

The PDU originated in an idea by three like-minded individuals – a manager, a nurse and a doctor. It has subsequently developed and continues to develop as a result of the hard work and determination of many people from all disciplines both within the clinical directorate and outside where a growing number of individuals recognise the potential benefits of the PDU ethos to patients.

Initiating the PDU necessitated a cultural change within the professional teams. The need to clarify roles and relationships was paramount to ensure that the skills of the team were used to maximum effect.

The breaking down of professional barriers and a positive approach to learning, not only within individual professional groups, but also as a multidisciplinary team, has been essential to the success of the PDU and will, I feel, continue to be important in the spreading of the concept across the organisation.

The PDU approach essentially stems from a belief within the multidisciplinary team (both clinical and non-clinical) that an approach to care management and delivery which is focused on patient need rather than professional and organisational priorities is essential to the provision of a high quality service.

I hope that my own and other members of the Steering Group's lead in setting the strategic direction of the PDU will demonstrate the commitment of the organisation to the need for a laboratory to test out theories about practice which will benefit the whole trust.

I believe we need to ensure that the PDU is integrated into the business planning processes of the organisation. My experience to date is that the unit's success is reliant on the commitment of its staff to explore and test new ideas with the aim of improving patient care. I firmly believe that this is being achieved.

One of my main priorities for the unit is to initiate an evaluation of its effectiveness using the skills of individuals outside the organisation to ensure we have an objective view of the work being carried out.

Conclusion

Since its inception, the PDU has striven to develop its staff and to involve them in developments within the unit. This has not always been easy against the continually changing organisational backdrop and ever-tighter resources at the clinical level.

Many individuals and groups have nevertheless maintained their enthusiasm and involvement throughout in spite of the tremendous pressures, and the team's dietitians and pharmacists, for example, have been particularly active and remain so in areas which have been supported by the PDU resources.

In November 1995, however, as a result of concerns about the mounting problems of maintaining the ethos of the PDU against an increasingly difficult backdrop – usually indifferent, at times hostile –

a questionnaire was sent to staff to obtain their views of the PDU. Of the 60 questionnaires sent 47 were returned. Of the staff questioned 60% had been in post more than a year. The aim of the survey was to get some idea of what people working on the original PDU wards understood the PDU to be and whether their views reflected those held by those who led the unit. Staff were asked a number of questions about their involvement and the level of support they received. There was consensus of opinion that staff were encouraged to suggest new approaches and to question practice. Most staff felt they were allowed to try out well-considered new ideas on PDU wards. The important features of a successful PDU were felt by the respondents to include high quality, multidisciplinary working, partnerships with patients and patient empowerment, continuous evaluation of practice which was researched based.

Interestingly, the majority of respondents did not appear to see the areas of research, staff development and career opportunities, value for money, clinical audit and partnerships with higher education as of equal importance to the unit. To some extent this perhaps reflects the primarily patient-based perspective of practitioners at ward and department level and was to be anticipated.

However, more seriously, just 25% of the staff questioned felt involved in PDU projects and there was no indication of any desire amongst the majority to become more involved. While there is no means of comparing this to other areas, it may well be on reflection that the engagement of 25% of practitioners at all levels within a multidisciplinary team in developmental work is beyond the level normally experienced in a clinical area. Nevertheless, the leaders of the unit were certainly disappointed with this outcome at the time, and clearly felt that this represented a downturn in the unit team's belief in itself as a result of the pressures arising from the latest hospital merger and its growing impact on the management of the hospital.

The PDU has been successful over a number of years in empowering staff to work together more effectively. A major focus has been on empowering the nursing staff who traditionally have been seen to provide 24 hour care which they may or may not have initiated. Primary nursing has proved to be a successful model to empower nursing staff and improve patient care.

Empowering other members of the multidisciplinary team has taken place on another level with a multidisciplinary team approach to all projects on the PDU. This responsibility has fallen to the PDU Leader and Research Practitioner to always ensure all disciplines are aware of the need to involve all their colleagues and include the patients' views where appropriate. The Clinical Forum and Clinical Audit have helped to support the dissemination of information across the disciplines as well as the teamwork.

The staff questionnaire shows that whilst the PDU has been successful in many ways, at the clinical level individuals often have difficulty in seeing a wider view beyond their practice areas and are easily discouraged by everyday pressures of work and by factors in the external environment from becoming involved in any developmental processes. To empower staff further it is essential that the PDU objectives are maintained as part of the business plan and are given a high profile by the organisation's managers or there is the potential in the future for the unit's work either to move further away from the wards and reflect less and less the real need of the patients, or to cease altogether. Staff can only be empowered and encouraged to become involved in the PDU process if the wider organisation is committed to empowering them and reinforces the message that their involvement in developing new practices for their patients and a preparedness to take measured risks in practice (and sometimes to fail) is something which the organisation finds acceptable and is prepared to actively support and reward.

Chapter 9
Patient empowerment

David Allsopp and Mike Lowry

After an explanation of the context within which empowerment as an idea has arisen, this chapter explains how the PDU seeks to empower patients and their families by encouraging greater participation in decision making, through health education and promotion and by providing more effective communication. Examples are provided of projects which support patient empowerment such as self-medication, developing an education programme for new diabetics based on their needs, the carers' support group, and use of lay diagnoses for patients. The need for a greater emphasis on empowering service users typified by the PDU approach is discussed in contrast with other approaches primarily focusing on empowering professionals.

Empowerment and the rise of consumerism

The issue of patient empowerment is one which has received a lot of attention in recent years, although since 1974 Community Health Councils have had a role in providing a voice for health service users. More recently there have general changes in society towards a more consumer-led culture: government policy has deliberately promoted ideas of individual rights, consumer choice and redress for poor quality goods or services. This is demonstrated by the launch of various consumer charters including the Patient's Charter for users of the NHS (DOH, 1995). In addition, the introduction of general management into the NHS has helped raise the profile of quality issues and of the need for consumer feedback. The Griffiths report of

1983 said that managers should 'ascertain how well the service is being delivered at local level by obtaining the experience and perceptions of patients and the community' (cited in Jones *et al.*, 1987, p. 7).

Management theory has also been heavily influenced by prominent authors such as Peters and Waterman (1982) who place the customer at the centre of efforts to succeed in business. An excellent company, they argue, asks customers what they want and gives it to them. Much effort has been expended in the NHS on seeking the views of patients and other users through satisfaction surveys. In nursing, the use of quality assessment tools such as Monitor (Goldstone *et al.*, 1984) has also drawn attention to the importance of finding out what patients think of their care, as well as to issues of process and record keeping. The use of audit has helped to develop a more questioning culture and has encouraged professionals from different disciplines to work together as medical and nursing audit has evolved into clinical audit.

All of these initiatives represent attempts by service providers to change the way in which service users are involved in the processes of care and treatment. All too often patients in hospital have been passive recipients of care delivered by professionals who assume they know best. Even the use of the term 'patient' signifies for some an unequal relationship with all the power being held by the professional.

At the same time that service providers are becoming more active in seeking users' views, the users themselves are becoming more proactive in asserting their wish to have more of a say about how health services are planned and delivered. Various patient interest groups have come into being over the years, usually focused on specific diseases, such as the Stroke Association, or with a more general focus such as the Patients' Association or the College of Health (Jones *et al.*, 1987).

In response to more knowledgeable and assertive patients, health services need to be committed to a more equal partnership between professional and patient. The use by some nurses of the term 'client' has become more common and maybe reflects a desire for a more equal relationship. Salvage (1992) describes how the Oxford Nursing Development Unit (NDU) talked of partnership thus:

> We listen to what the patient has to say and through . . . communication
> . . . we help him to become clear on his concerns around (his) particular
> treatment plan . . . he will clarify his own motivations.

> The nurses will aim to work in such a way that the patient becomes a
> partner who is actively encouraged to become an equal voice in deci-
> sion making about his nursing and other therapies (p. 13).

The fact that nurses and others are using words like partnership to
describe their relationship with patients is interesting and seemingly
appealing, but it is not clear that much has really changed in the
health service generally.

What is meant by 'empowerment'?

Chapter 8 has already dealt with the ways in which the PDU seeks to
empower staff. In the PDU the term empowerment relates to both
staff and patients and is seen as the transfer of power over decisions.
Within the PDU this means the devolution of power 'downwards'
through the organisation. This is partly because of conscious decisions by managers to give more responsibility to those such as ward
sisters, and also because of the loss of middle layers of management
which have necessitated such a transfer of responsibility. In order
that patients can be empowered, those working with them also have
to have to be empowered. The introduction of primary nursing and
a ward sister development programme are examples of ways in
which staff were empowered. The inclusion in various projects of
staff from all disciplines who were not used to such involvement also
did much to empower them. The work described in Chapter 6 on
the multidisciplinary patient assessment documentation illustrates
how nurses were empowered by being able to make referrals to therapists without needing a doctor's signature. The other key aspect of
empowerment, whether of staff or patients, is education. As stated in
Chapter 2, the PDU placed a heavy emphasis on providing opportunities for staff development and training. Using such means as
project-based learning, mentorship and learning contracts, the PDU
was able to support staff in the development of their skills so that they
could participate fully in debates about practice.

The first statement in the PDU philosophy statement is that

> we believe that patients have the right to be involved in decisions about
> their care and that we should work towards empowering them fully.

It must be said that such a statement does not fit with the prevailing
NHS ethos, which is more to do with organising and delivering
services according to professionals' perceptions of what is required.
This does not mean that services are totally insensitive to users' needs,
but that, as much of the knowledge of disease and its treatment

lies with professionals, then the power over decisions also lies with them. Consequently, any attempt to involve users in decisions about their care must depend upon them becoming much more knowledgeable.

The PDU has right from the start sought to involve service users more in decision making. A range of means has been used, including surveys to seek views about such issues as mixed sex wards, the use of day room areas, satisfaction with nursing care, visitors' satisfaction and smoking. Projects which involve giving more information to patients and relatives include self-medication, diabetes education, cardiac rehabilitation and the carers' support group. Efforts to encourage greater participation by patients in decision making have included walk round reports involving patients, asking patients to comment on care plans, the use of patient-held records and a project to provide written information in lay terms concerning diagnoses and treatment.

Although such projects demonstrate promising development towards more empowered users, there are two important points to be made:

- Credit must by given to those professionals of all disciplines who spend a great deal of time and energy explaining, educating and in the promotion of independence, involving patients and their carers in complex decisions.
- Despite such efforts and those mentioned previously as PDU projects, there is still a long way to go before fully empowered users are the norm rather than the exception. Many patients in hospital remain blissfully ignorant of decision making processes and are happy to stay that way. They have complete trust in the professional when on occasion a little scepticism would be useful, and there is a lack of assertiveness about wanting to have a greater say which can lead professionals to mistakenly believe that consent is granted. More knowledgeable and assertive patients provide a considerable challenge to professionals, who are then forced into a direct accountability which some find uncomfortable. This trend seems likely to continue, as new generations of patient come forward who are less willing to be passive than those who came before.

This chapter continues by describing four projects:

- the self-medication project referred to in Chapter 7

- a project aimed at developing the education provided for those recently diagnosed as having diabetes
- a carers' support group
- a project to provide patients with information on diagnosis and treatment using lay terminology.

Self-medication

This piece of research (described in more detail in Chapter 7) was conducted in the PDU by a pharmacist and a nurse and funded by a grant from the regional health authority (Lowe *et al.*, 1995). The aim was to test whether patients going through an inpatient self-medication programme performed better on assessments of knowledge and compliance with prescription than a similar group going through standard preparation before discharge.

Briefly, the results showed that the patients going through the self-medication 'treatment' performed significantly better on knowledge and compliance after discharge than the control group.

The benefits of self-medication in empowering patients included:

- autonomy
- independence during and after discharge
- self-respect
- option of taking medicines to suit patients' own needs and plans for day
- better preparation for discharge.

Thinking back to the definition of empowerment as a transfer of power, it becomes clear that involving patients in a self-medication project is an effective way of giving them much greater control in a way which shows respect for their right to self-determination. Being able to take your own tablets to suit your own timetable and needs is how people expect to behave at home, so why not in hospital too? To take such control away unnecessarily to suit the system seems almost to be insulting to people's abilities. The common hospital approach of nurses doing medicine rounds and spending two minutes 'explaining' medication just before discharge is totally inadequate in preparing patients for dealing with their medicines. As well as empowering patients during their hospital stay, self-medication sustains the empowerment after discharge. By providing support through education and practice in hospital, treatment regimes can be administered much more accurately after discharge, with consequent benefits of more effective treatment. In addition, by educating patients about their medicines and why they are necessary, patients become more knowledgeable about their diseases than they might otherwise have done.

Educational provision for those recently diagnosed as having diabetes

Traditional approaches in the NHS to the education of people newly diagnosed with diabetes has focused upon the role of GPs and more recently practice nurses, and hospital outpatient departments. There has also been an increase in the provision in specialist departments/centres which provide a resource to those with diabetes. The value of education programmes lies in the prevention of acute complications such as foot disease and eye problems, which are highly treatable and preventable (McColl and Gulliford, 1993). In a study of 10 000 patients, Davidson (1983) showed that a comprehensive diabetes care programme with evaluation, education, therapy and follow-up significantly reduced diabetic ketoacidosis.

In the PDU the concern was how to give patients with newly diagnosed diabetes a much greater say over what they needed to be educated about and how. By asking them to tell us directly what they needed it was hoped that they would be better empowered in taking control of their health and maintaining their independence as long as possible.

There was also a desire to develop the skills of staff in the PDU, by involving them in research for the first time, by providing opportunities to talk directly with patients about their needs for teaching, and by enabling them to influence educational provision for those with newly diagnosed diabetes.

Building on an initial idea from a senior lecturer at a local university, a collaborative research project was developed with the aim of seeking the views of those recently diagnosed as having diabetes about their experiences of the NHS in meeting their needs to learn about diabetes and how to cope with it. A primary nurse was seconded to the project part time as research assistant. Her replacement on the ward was funded through the (small) study leave budget. A learning contract was agreed between the nurse, her ward sister and the PDU leader. The seconded nurse gained some insight into the education patients received at their first hospital visit through her observations in outpatients. Patients often seemed confused by the information they had been given, and there seemed to be considerable scope for reviewing their difficulties.

In designing the study it was agreed that there was a need to start from the beginning and ask the subjects what they thought, with no preconceptions of what they might say (Lowry, 1995a). The aims of the study were to find out what people newly diagnosed as having diabetes and their close relatives thought they needed to know to help them cope with the demands of having diabetes, and to develop educational provision to better meet the needs of people with this condition.

The most productive way of doing this was thought to be the use of a focus group. Holloway and Wheeler (1996) describe a focus group as involving

> a number of people with common experiences or characteristics who are interviewed by a researcher . . . for the purpose of eliciting ideas, thoughts and perceptions about a specific topic or certain issues linked to an area of interest (p. 144).

Focus groups were first used in the 1920s and have been popular with market researchers ever since. In a health care context a focus group can help to evaluate services, and has the advantage over other types of evaluation in that perspectives other than those identified by the researcher can be identified. In the PDU the interest was in having an open mind about the sort of issues of concern to people with newly diagnosed diabetes. Arranging a focus group of those newly diagnosed as having diabetes and including in the group, if they wished, a close relative, was seen as a productive way of generating a wealth of data about the service provided. Alternatively, some sort of postal survey or a series of one-to-one interviews might have been conducted. A postal survey at this stage was rejected as the researchers did not want to pre-judge (by their selection of questions) what issues might be important to these individuals. Using a focus group allowed for a concentrated effort in data gathering, rich in detail and productive of ideas. There was also a desire to gain experience of the focus group approach to see if it would be useful in other situations.

A group of eight recent patients and relatives were invited to express their views and they agreed to follow up interviews at home to explore the data further. Potential participants were identified from lists of referrals to the hospital. Medical case notes were examined to confirm diagnosis. Prospective participants were invited by letter to attend and both the focus group and interviews were tape recorded (with consent) and the transcripts analysed using Burnard's method of content analysis (Burnard, 1991). The study aimed to use the data as a basis for review of the existing diabetic education provision and for further quantitative research to establish the extent of problems identified in representative groups of similar subjects. The focus group meeting was scheduled to last for one and a half hours (it actually lasted two and a half), and was facilitated by one of the researchers, using a prepared schedule as a guide. Participants were also encouraged to speak about whatever was important to them. Four of the group participants were able to take part in follow-up interviews.

Data analysis

Tape recordings of the focus group and interviews were transcribed and subjected to content analysis to identify themes.

The findings

The analysis of the focus group transcript identified seven main themes, which are set out in Table 9.1. The themes covered a wide range of experiences, starting before diagnosis was made, becoming ill and making first contact with the NHS, expressing views of information provided, the reaction of group participants to their diagnosis, the support they received and their anxieties and fears for the future.

Table 9.1 Themes identified from focus group analysis

Symptoms and experiences pre-diagnosis
Information provision
Reaction to diagnosis
Support after diagnosis
Anxieties and fears for the future (physical issues)
Anxieties and fears for the future (psycho-social issues)
Diet and lifestyle changes

Theme 1: Symptoms and experiences pre-diagnosis

None of the group seemed to understand what was happening to them when their signs and symptoms first appeared. Feeling faint, feeling stressed, being sick with vomiting, drinking a lot of liquid, weight loss and having flu-like symptoms were all described by one or another. There was a desire to explain these experiences but participants found themselves unable to do this. None realised they had diabetes. One had collapsed and had woken up in hospital, while others had just gone to their GP who had made the diagnosis. Misconceptions were sometimes apparent. One woman with a leg ulcer thought the ulcer had caused the diabetes. Another thought that the heart problems for which she was being treated were linked to the diabetes. Another thought her postnatal depression in earlier years was explained by the diabetes associated with pregnancy.

Theme 2: Information provision

All group members had admitted to a great deal of ignorance about diabetes and how to live with it, and a sense of frustration with the professionals they came into contact with.

One group member said

> I feel very frustrated because I have just recently had my appointment at this hospital to see a consultant and I was here for an hour and I saw him for three minutes, and I have only been diagnosed for a few months, I was totally ignorant about the condition itself.

Some had found advice from professionals helpful, while others had not. Two participants had found dietitians very supportive, with one saying that 'she wrote me a diet out, I've been fit as anything, much more fit than before, very active'. Another commented 'when I was asked if I wanted to see a dietitian last time, I said I thought it would be a waste of time'. There was a desire for some sort of system which would guide them in their decisions over what to eat and what to leave out of their diet. There was also a request for more guidance on sites of injection. Finally, there was some admission that participants still did not know what diabetes really was: 'I still don't know what it means'. One thought her leg ulcer had caused her diabetes.

Theme 3: Reaction to diagnosis

What came across strongly from the group was the profound sense of shock experienced after being told of their diagnosis. Statements like these were typical:

> I was shattered. I really was very shocked
> (I felt) disbelief that this could be happening to yourself
> I knew what my father was like when he was diabetic, he was aggressive and fits of hysteria that he had, even though I knew all that and I knew I had it before and it was said flippantly, 'you did expect this didn't you?', it was again still quite a shock.

For some there was the hope that somehow things would right themselves:

> Part of me believed that it was some kind of strange metabolic blip and after a week or so I wouldn't need the insulin was my feeling. Now they obviously didn't think that because they then arrived with a syringe and

> an orange to practise on and I injected this orange, then two days later I injected myself. I think even when I left hospital I still thought my physiology would re-establish itself.

Soon the realisation dawned that their lives would never be the same:

> So in my case a time has to come when I admit to myself 'no I am going to have to do this for the rest of my life'. I suppose that is my main memory of the transition from being so called ordinary to so called diabetic.

Another said

> It is very difficult, you have a pattern of life for so many years, it's very difficult to suddenly rethink the way in which you have to approach life and in which way you have to eat. Everything in your life in fact, even fitting in time to test your blood, I find that very difficult, when I do it at work, it's very difficult. All that has to be re-thought, you have to sit back and analyse your own feelings about it as well, it's hard to sit back, I just haven't been able to do that really. I need someone to talk to and sort my own head out really about it.

For one, the feeling that the diabetes had been diagnosed and was being treated was reassuring:

> I feel so safe that I am in here and that they have diagnosed something and I am being sorted out.

Theme 4: Support after diagnosis

There were mixed views of the support given by health service professionals after diagnosis. Comments critical of the time available to see the consultant in out patients were made, tempered by an understanding of why this might be:

> You walk into outpatients once (every) four months and you walk out again and you never speak to anyone except a nurse who says 'hold your finger out' or 'this can't be the correct reading for your weight.'

There were mixed statements about support from dietitians, more positive than negative, and there was also a feeling that professionals could do more:

> The fact that health professions, people caring for those with diabetes they very often focus on certain aspects of the condition, but maybe don't realise what other things are affecting you, and what your concerns are.

As well as blaming herself for failing to stick to her diet, one participant highlighted support as an issue:

There is so much more that can be done to help people, and I feel that one of the reasons is because I haven't had support. . . . I really feel there is nothing there behind us to hold us up. . . . There needs to be some kind of support, even if it's only some kind of counter of some kind that is available for you to pop into if you come in for an appointment at the hospital.

One participant had a dog which had also developed diabetes. The vet was said to be very helpful:

We had more information about the dog's diabetes, we had a video, we had long explanations, we had telephone numbers to ring up in case we got into difficulties.

Themes 5 and 6: Anxieties and fears for the future

One of the results of becoming more knowledgeable about diabetes is the realisation of what might go wrong in the future. Some group participants had learned of the possibilities from relatives with diabetes or from friends and neighbours also having the disease. Comments included:

I supposed I was concerned, very concerned in the sense I knew what had happened to members of my family who had it and I knew it was linked to other disorders.

My condition is going to be getting worse all the time. I know it's worsening, it's getting worse now because I haven't been able to keep to the diet, I feel as though I don't know what is happening to me, I know I have this daunting feel that things are getting worse all the time.

My sister had it. The danger was that she nearly lost a leg, but she died quite suddenly. This is at the back of your mind and is a bit frightening you see.

Attempts are made to link what has been explained by professionals to what is known from experience:

I have a next door neighbour who I know has diabetes and he was having this problem with his feet, and again this was explained to me when I was diagnosed I had to be very careful with my feet. I didn't know why I had to be careful with my feet.

Other anxieties concerned fears about the development of the condition and how it might affect them, and concerns about how relatives might be affected also. Living alone also caused concern, in case anything went wrong and no one knew. Personal experience of deaths in the family related to diabetes heightened anxieties still further.

Themes 7 : Diet and lifestyle changes

Diet figured largely in the comments of group members. Diabetes obviously has a profound effect on the need to rethink dietary habits and to consider necessary changes to lifestyle:

I think diabetes is a condition which comes upon you very suddenly. You have to re-examine your whole work schedule, your whole diet, you have to re-examine everything.

Diabetes also causes considerable fear in some:

After being diagnosed diabetic I was absolutely terrified to eat anything.

After a while, the fear turns to a sort of resignation:

When I was first diagnosed I was going around the supermarket looking up ingredients on every single packet, to analyse if there was any sugar in this, whether it was a tin or packet. Now I don't bother, I just bung it all in and I don't think about it.

The message that seemed to be coming across was that adapting to dietary changes was difficult, and the advice and information given by professionals was either too generalised or was not taken in by patients. Difficulties with sticking to recommended diets were often described, as well as problems with maintaining body weight at appropriate levels. The process of learning to adapt to such changes was problematical for some, such as the participant who said

I am struggling badly because I am on a diet that is not working for me and I work under a great deal of stress all the time.

Everyone appeared to know that they needed to be careful about their sugar intake, though not all managed this. They also knew that the amount of exercise they took was relevant. There was puzzlement that they could eat the same things every day and exercise by the same amount and yet measure differing blood sugar levels. They knew about the need to stop smoking, to lose weight, and to look after their feet. Changing the teachings of childhood was difficult for some:

When I was little I was also told eat up, eat up, don't leave anything.

Diabetes education and empowerment

What seems to come across from the focus group discussion is a sense of loss of control over one's body and lifestyle. There is immense frustration at not being able to carry on as before and becoming dependent on the health care system. The way in which the group developed feelings of disempowerment is nicely illustrated thus:

Something that has come out before is the feeling of not being in control; that something has happened either to yourself or to someone that you are close to and the control is given to somebody else to deal with it . . . all your life you are the one who makes the decisions and very soon you find yourself in a position where somehow you lose that ability, and I think it seems very important to be able to take hold of the situation again and to have some say and control and to have some understanding and knowledge rather than giving it to somebody else to make the decisions for you.

The findings of the focus group study suggest various problems with the ways in which newly diagnosed adults are helped in adapting to the demands placed on them. If the findings of this study are representative of most people with diabetes, there needs to be a review of diabetes education, at least at a local level. In order that people with diabetes can regain a sense of control over their lives consideration needs to be given to ways of achieving this. Certainly it seems that very careful, repeated explanations are needed, which overturn some of the misconceptions people sometimes have, such as the lady who thought her diabetes was caused by her leg ulcer. It may be that such explanations are already provided, and that they are not taken in. Why is this? Is it because opportunities for education are too infrequent, so that patients forget what has been said? One of the difficulties must be that the potential for variation in diet between people is enormous, so providing specific advice is problematic. People need to learn principles which they can interpret to suit their own specific needs. Perhaps they also need to learn, through experience, how to relate the principles to their own circumstances. They need to take risks (which they undoubtedly do anyway) and reflect on what works and what does not. The problem is that such risk taking can be dangerous, even life threatening, so support is needed in providing advice when it is needed, not weeks later in outpatients.

For the PDU the challenge now is what to do with these findings from the diabetes study. A qualitative study such as this is very productive in generating data about a small group of people with a shared problem. The next task is to find out how typical these findings are of the experience of more representative groups. Although the findings can raise questions about the nature and content of diabetes education which will undoubtedly inform the practice of individuals, it would be premature to change the service as a whole without further research to corroborate these initial findings.

A truly empowered person with diabetes would be knowledgeable about the disease, its treatment and its likely course, would know how to cope with variations in signs and symptoms and would know where to seek help and advice if needed. Professionals have a responsibility to provide such support, which is, because of the nature of diabetes, a multidisciplinary issue. The PDU provides a model of how such issues can be dealt with. The findings will be discussed at a multidisciplinary meeting and plans for further research and action to respond to the issues taken. One way forward is to offer regular opportunities to new diabetics for meeting to discuss with knowledgeable experts (including other people with diabetes) ways of dealing with the problems faced. In the focus group meeting there was a lot of support for this idea. One participant said (and the others agreed)

> I found it very helpful to meet people in a similar position and it's been the first glimmer of light that I have had since I was diagnosed being a diabetic in December last year. I think something of this kind should have happened then.

The carers' support group

Another example of ways in which the PDU sought to empower users of the medical services was by means of the carers' support group. This was established by primary nurse Irene Waddington and social worker Margaret Buckle. They were particularly concerned with the issue of carer strain, which they were very familiar with in their work with older patients in the PDU and previously at St George's Hospital. The sorts of difficulties faced by carers include exhaustion and depression, as they often struggle alone to look after a family member for extended periods of time, often years. Feelings of anger at being taken for granted by the person for whom they are caring, and at those who could help but do not, are common. Social life is often non-existent and carers have limited knowledge of what help is available or where to seek assistance.

Carers of patients on one PDU ward were offered the opportunity to participate in the support group. Its aims are to provide information on such things as benefit availability and application procedures, the development of skills such as moving and handling of people with a disability, the use of aids and adaptations, the use of devices for dealing with medication problems, advice on diet and healthy eating and information about specific diseases such as stroke. A wide range of professionals have assisted with carers' group sessions, including physiotherapists, occupational therapists, pharmacists, dietitians, doctors and Benefits Agency staff.

The benefits of involvement in the group are clear. Carers are much better able to cope, knowing they have somewhere to go to meet with others in a similar position. Problems are shared and ideas exchanged for dealing with them. Just getting out of the house is something valued very highly, and meetings are much looked forward to.

Patient information project

The following account by Dr Chris Patterson, Senior Registrar in Geriatrics in the PDU, describes a project aimed at assessing what elderly patients could remember about their diagnosis and whether or not written information improves recall. This was a randomised study, with patients receiving either a written information sheet at the time of their discharge or standard care (controls). Patients were then contacted two weeks after discharge and all completed a questionnaire about their diagnosis.

Patient satisfaction

The need for hospital care providers to improve the quality of care for patients has been highlighted by the Patient's Charter and the NHS reviews. Patient satisfaction is important to providers of health care, and managers must now plan services to reflect the patients' needs. Satisfaction of the patient may correlate with outcome of treatment, compliance with treatment and follow-up, and possibly even litigation.

Many factors are involved in the perception of care:

- communication skills of the care provider
- convenience and outcome of treatment
- the environment in which care is delivered.

Studies have shown that the amount of information given to patients about medical care improves satisfaction in a variety of settings including paediatrics, emergency departments, general medical wards as well as in the use of prescription information leaflets.

Measuring patient satisfaction can be difficult: direct questions about satisfaction tend to encourage positive responses and hence would be viewed with caution as they may hide problems which exist. It has been suggested that asking patients detailed questions about what happened during their stay in hospital will highlight problems of care that would not have been shown by standard general questions about satisfaction.

Patient information

Many strategies have been put forward to avoid the problems of patient dissatisfaction and poor compliance caused by inadequate communication. The trend has been towards both patient education and the provision of written and other information for patients to try and improve recall and understanding of medical information. The Department of Health has stated that patients and relatives should be fully informed before discharge from hospital and that important pieces of information, particularly with regard to medication, should be provided in written form.

Evidence suggests patients want more information about all aspects of their medical care. However, when information is given orally, much of it is incompletely understood and often quickly forgotten, and thus patients are keen to receive written information, particularly with respect to treatment (Lowry, 1995b). Written information should improve knowledge and recall in order to be of value. Previous studies suggest that written information does indeed increase knowledge and level of compliance, although effects on outcome are less impressive. However, recall of medical information does not seem to be improved by written information. Psychological literature has suggested that information provided should be 'concrete' and that use of videotaped information and specific examples may be very effective. Of course there may be considerable differences in the way patients digest information, and it may be that different versions of information sheets should be available so that patients can choose a level of information which can best suit their behaviour and needs. The readability of written information is important since many information sheets have proved too difficult for the majority of adult readers.

Elderly patients, often with multiple diagnoses and possible communication difficulties, may have particular problems recalling information. Patterson and Teale (1997) studied patients (mean age 75 years) discharged from an acute medical elderly ward and showed that patient recall of information regarding diagnosis was poor but was significantly improved by providing simple written information at discharge. In addition, patients receiving written information were significantly more satisfied with information received than the control group who received standard care.

Patient views

In order to assess what elderly patients could recall about their diagnosis and whether or not written information improves recall, consecutive patients discharged from one acute ward (general medicine with an interest in the elderly) were studied. Patients were randomised to receive either a written information sheet at the time of their discharge or standard care (controls). They were then contacted two weeks after discharge and all completed a questionnaire about their diagnosis. The majority responded to the first mailing of the questionnaire and most of the remainder to the second, with just two patients responding to a visit to their home. Experience suggests the elderly often have a high response rate to such questionnaires.

Only one third of control patients correctly recalled their diagnosis compared with almost two thirds of those given an information sheet (p <0.05). Despite poor recall, three quarters of control patients were satisfied with information given although this rose significantly with the provision of an information sheet.

Patient quotes

During the study, patients were invited to write down both the main illness for which they were recently treated in hospital, and a list of all other medical problems. Examples of answers deemed to be correct are given in Table 9.2.

Other quotes (interestingly from patients who did not recall their diagnosis correctly) included:

> The care and information on the ward could not have been better. My thanks to all concerned.
> Please accept a cheque in appreciation of my stay.

Table 9.2 Examples of answers deemed to be correct or incorrect

Correct answer	diagnosis
High blood pressure	Hypertension
Wear and tear arthritis	Osteoarthritis
Blood clot on lung	Pulmonary embolus
Narrowed heart valve	Aortic stenosis
Irregular heart beat	Atrial fibrillation
Incorrect answer	
Difficulty breathing	Chest infection
Water trouble	Heart failure
Bad heart	Angina
Stiff leg	Stroke

Empowering patients and empowering professionals

There is a difference in emphasis between the PDU and the NDU approach. The latter is based on a belief that by empowering nurses 'one creates the opportunities to empower patients' (Evans, 1992). There is no disagreement about this point between PDU and NDU approaches. If anything, the PDU extends the principle to other professionals and to the team. Empowered individuals function more effectively within teams and teams also become more effective. Empowered professionals can empower patients but this should not be taken for granted. The PDU makes a particular point of seeking to empower patients, recognising that this can only happen if professionals are empowered also, and are willing and able to transfer power to patients.

Conclusion

The projects presented in this chapter provide examples of a range of different approaches to empowering patients in the PDU. The threads common to all the projects described in this chapter are the provision of accessible information as a means of empowerment and a genuine underlying desire to involve the users of the service, beyond the level of mere tokenism. The more knowledgeable service users become, the more empowered they can be. One can only make free and rational choices if one has access to information. Not all choose to exercise their sense of empowerment fully, nor does the seeking of information necessarily correlate with a desire to participate fully in decision-making processes (Marks, 1993).

As long as professionals control information and how much they choose to tell patients and others, there will always be an unequal relationship. The PDU has, in good faith, made serious attempts to bridge the gap between professional and patient, but it is recognised that there is still some way to go before there is a truly empowered client group. The sort of changes discussed involve a considerable shift in thinking by all concerned, not just in health care, but in society at large. A truly democratic society educates its members to make their own decisions and choices, including those made in the provision of health care. The PDU has made a small but significant contribution towards achieving this aim.

Chapter 10
Networking for
innovation

Steve Page

A dictionary definition of a network is 'a group of persons sharing an aim, interest, etc., and frequently communicating with or helping each other'. The idea of creating a network or of 'networking' with other people or groups is frequently used in the health service and in broad terms the benefits of linking up with others to share ideas and information are well accepted. An NHS booklet has even been published as part of the Opportunity 2000 initiative, which extols the virtues of such activity (NHS Executive, 1994).

However, frequently the reason for such activity and its specific aims and objectives are not well explored and the perception can arise of networking activity as a 'trendy' aimless activity from which only a privileged few derive personal benefit and enjoyment. In the meantime, the majority of the workforce remains unaffected, and no impact on quality of care given to patients is detectable.

Negative impact of networking

Previous chapters have commented on the danger for development units of being perceived as elitist. In many ways this is one of the ways in which this perception can be most powerfully fuelled. Access – to travel, other organisations, local and national events, key figures, for example – can be seen as a significant reward. Where these rewards are not perceptibly linked to actions or benefits in the organisation, this can rapidly lead to disillusionment and a deep scepticism among the remainder of the workforce who feel excluded. An impression is given of the development of exclusive coteries engaged in esoteric debates about issues of no direct benefit to anyone in the practice setting.

Religiously feeding back on such events and discussions to the remainder of the team on one's return is likely, of course, not to diminish this perception but to magnify it further. Once this feeling takes hold, the disillusionment and scepticism in the team can become inversely related to the enthusiasm and commitment of the networkers. The more exciting the events and debates and the more innovative the ideas fed back to the team, the less engaged they become by the whole process. This response to networking in a development unit can, of course, develop at a variety of levels – within the unit itself, across an organisation, or on a regional or national scale.

In addition to this, networking can be an enormously resource-intensive activity. It demands both money and time, for travel and for work related to planning and subsequent activities. Where the network is focused on development of specific ideas or practices, it can also be seen to be grossly inefficient and slow in progressing, contributing to the increased complexity of communication and co-ordination of an activity compared with similar work focused solely within the organisation. This is exacerbated by the frequently poor access to information technology within the clinical setting.

This being the case, networking can represent a serious dilution of the resources and energy available to carry out work within a unit – both to support the continued development of the unit's culture for change and to promote tangible new developments and their uptake in practice. As has been argued in previous chapters, in most organisations the continued survival of a development unit is dependent on its ability to demonstrate its contribution to the achievement of the organisation's goals.

The advent of NHS trusts has resulted in predominantly inward-looking organisations, for whom broader NHS-wide and long-term benefits are of less relevance than those which are short-term, local and organisation-specific. Dilution of the resources targeted within the organisation can therefore be a dangerous practice for a development unit, with obvious potential consequences.

These negative aspects of networking have been deliberately set out at the start of this chapter, because they are frequently hidden and unrecognised or unacknowledged in the generally rosy view of the activity. Of course, this is not to imply a lack of belief in the potential benefits of networking both to the unit and, via the PDU, to the organisation as a whole. In fact, the activity is an integral part of the PDU's philosophy and style of working, from both the micro level of networking between disciplines within the team and the macro levels of networking across the hospital and between organisations – with other NHS trusts, universities, research units, for example.

Later parts of this chapter will seek to define in more detail some of the specific benefits gained by the PDU and others through networking activity. However, first it is important to consider in general terms how the PDU approached the activity of networking in order to be able to increase its benefits, without falling into the traps outlined above.

Approach to networking in the PDU

Within the PDU, the activity of networking is not a haphazard, vaguely positive exercise. Rather, it is implicit in the unit's philosophy and aims – the elements of which have been defined and periodically reviewed by the whole team.

An emphasis on patient focus, as has been argued earlier, encourages practitioners to cross narrow professional boundaries within the unit, but also fosters a broader perspective in addressing patient care issues beyond the boundaries of the immediate organisation. The multidisciplinary emphasis promotes inclusion of different perspectives both from within the unit and beyond, rather than excluding them. The drive to develop research activity within the unit and to evaluate its developments leads its team naturally to develop partnerships with other care providers and with academic research units. The enormous emphasis on development of staff as a means of changing culture and fuelling development of quality patient care can only be brought to fruition through the development of strong partnerships between the PDU and educationalists, and through exposure of staff to new or different experiences and ideas.

Finally, if the *raison d'être* of the PDU is to share its ideas and work with other areas, to bring about maximum benefits from its activities, then a positive and open approach to communication with others is essential. This must begin with the development of effective networks at home within the host organisation, but will not stop at these boundaries – the philosophy of the PDU is consistent with that of a health service, rather than of distinct care providers.

The first important point, then, is that networking is seen to relate to the underlying philosophy of the unit and it is from here that it draws its specific objectives. For this reason, networking in the PDU has always been perceived to be the province of any member of the team, from any discipline at any grade, rather than that of a few chosen practitioners.

The second important principle underlying the PDU's approach to networking develops this further. Sharing a philosophy and broad aims is probably sufficient to stimulate the beginning of a network. It will enable people to share ideas and concerns and to learn from one another on a personal level. It would be possible to set free the whole staff of a unit to seek out connections and form partnerships at will, and each individual would almost certainly gain from the exercise and some benefit might even be brought back to the unit itself and to its patients. However, having a shared philosophy and broad aims may not, in themselves, be sufficient to enable us to derive the maximum benefit from the activity.

Some individuals may be unable to see a benefit in an activity not linked to practice, or may not readily be able to pick out potential partners who would further the development of their own thoughts or practice. Others may enjoy the activity, but not make the connection between the pleasure of travelling or meeting new people and any learning to be gained. Finally, and most commonly, networking itself can be positive, well-received and felt to benefit individuals involved, but to have no obvious outlet in terms of practical developments within the unit. In these respects, networking is probably no different from any educational activity. It differs only in that the intangibility of the process as compared to formal educational activities makes the widely acknowledged difficulty of linking education to practice even tougher than usual.

The second central element of the PDUs approach to networking, therefore, is to balance the freedom of access of any in the team to networking activity, with the tying in of any such activity to specific objectives within the unit. These objectives may relate to specific developmental project work, to a research study, to the development of education programmes, to the sharing with others of areas of work to which the practitioner has previously contributed, or to personal development objectives. In any event, the specific purpose and expected outcomes of the network are defined in advance and therefore can be seen to relate to the objectives and philosophy of the PDU and organisation as a whole.

This gives clear objectives to the leaders of the activity, but also specifically enables members of the team, who might normally find networking an intangible exercise and difficult to relate to practice, to see direct connections. This acts both as a strong motivator and also facilitates a more focused approach to the exercise – i.e. it helps people to look at the right things, ask the right questions, think directly about what and how issues might be applicable to their own practice. It also enables the PDU to evaluate much more effectively the real benefits to its team and, of course, to patient care of the resources committed to any specific networking activity.

The facilitation of these connections between the PDU's overall strategy and specific project objectives and networking with other individuals and organisations forms a considerable part of the roles of PDU Leader and of its Research Practitioner. Their roles are to maximise both the depth of focus towards specific issues on the unit's agenda and the breadth of access among different practitioners within the multidisciplinary team. A good example of this is the development of the unit's Research Advisory Group (RAG). This group, described in detail in Chapter 7, was established to provide access for practitioners within the unit to wide-ranging research expertise, where previously this had been entirely unavailable. To start, specific links were made with individuals in a number of organisations and with a variety of skills and backgrounds. A regular meeting of these individuals was convened so that practitioners could access them directly for advice about their proposed research-related activity.

More recently as such advice has become more readily available through academic courses and other professional channels, a more flexible approach has been developed, whereby the network of contacts has been broadened and advice and support are facilitated on a more individualised basis by the Research Practitioner and PDU Leader.

Another function of the PDU Leader and Research Practitioner is to facilitate a broader base for networking than is the norm among most professionals. Most commonly, networking activity takes place along markedly uniprofessional lines. Doctors network with other doctors, physiotherapists with physiotherapists and nurses with nurses. The ethos of the PDU blows this approach wide open, encouraging any interested person to network with any other whatever their background. The Leader and Research Practitioner, with their multidisciplinary remits, support and facilitate this.

Potential benefits of networking

Having highlighted some of the pitfalls and negative outcomes of networking, what then are its potential benefits?

To the PDU, the following benefits were identified:

- Broadening the base of knowledge and information to apply to a subject of interest to the unit – working on the very basic principle that two (or more) minds are better than one.
- Import from other areas of ideas either new to the unit or developed in a different direction. Such ideas provide valuable stimuli for new developments, and also, when these ideas are from within the PDU's host organisation, help to dispel the negative image of the unit as elitist and evangelistic.
- The potential to combine resources in order to exert greater influence or political leverage on an issue. Such combinations might be within the organisation, between organisations, (hospital – hospital, hospital – community, hospital – university, hospital – research unit) or between professions.
- Potential to combine (as above) to solve a problem. A good example of this was the link forged between PDU and mental health NDU (part of the local Community and Mental Health Trust) described in detail below.
- Concentration of resources (financial or personnel) available to address an issue by combining efforts of various organisations.
- Increasing the potential to draw in resources from outside funding agencies by demonstrating multiagency collaboration and consensus.
- Increasing the credibility of a development by demonstrating its value to a number of agencies.
- Increasing the applicability of PDU developments by collaborating with others in their implementation and evaluation.
- Increasing awareness of the complexity of relevant issues, as a means to overcome practitioners' 'political naivety'.
- Derivation of mutual but differing benefits, eg. hospital – hospital, hospital – university, service – research. A useful example of this is the mutual benefit to be gained by collaboration between the hospital and a research unit. A joint project which did not come to fruition (for practical reasons related to the difficulty of finding a comparable unit for research purposes), between the PDU and York University, was of significant benefit to the unit because of the potential to have its impact formally evaluated by a well respected and objective research team. Its benefits to the unit also included the level of research expertise this collaboration would bring into contact with its staff; and the credibility and kudos this connection would bring to the unit both internally with its own

Trust executives and externally. To the research unit, benefits included the chance to forge a formal collaboration with a local provider unit, and to be involved in an evaluation study which was unique and which appeared to address, in an innovative way, one of the national priorities related to clinical effectiveness and multidisciplinary practice.

- The increase of breadth of input to smaller disciplines within a hospital. For example, some of the therapy disciplines within any given care team can consist of only a handful of individuals. Their pool of new ideas may therefore be relatively narrow and the potential for stasis is high. Contacts with other professionals within these disciplines either from other service providers or from academia can only enrich the team's ideas.

- Similarly, opening the breadth of contacts to other disciples serves to enrich the ideas and practices of the whole multidisciplinary team within the unit. Sometimes, within a given unit, some disciplines are more innovative and dominant than others. Exposure to other areas where innovative ideas and leadership are supplied by a different discipline both gives confidence to the underdogs and allows the leading disciplines to understand their potential contribution more readily.

- Increasing the range of the PDU's contacts enables it to build personal links between key individuals and effective working partnerships which will facilitate the sharing and dissemination of its ideas. The development of respect and rapport between individuals in this context is vital and it is unlikely that practice will be developed in a collaborative way without them.

- The development of increased interest and excitement within the PDU team by exposure to other ideas and experiences.

- Networking can be seen as a reward for hard work or good ideas, while continuing to promote these qualities and encouraging further development within the unit.

Examples of networking within the PDU

Networking within the PDU operates on a number of levels – within the unit's multidisciplinary team itself, between the PDU and other areas of its host organisation, and between the PDU and other organisations.

The first two of these spheres of activity have been described in detail in other chapters and therefore this section concentrates primarily on the third. It is not uncommon for developmental units to find it difficult to be prophets in their own land, while enjoying considerable reputations and successes outside. Some of the reasons for this relate to issues discussed at the start of this chapter. Probably, this is exacerbated by the adoption of primarily information giving, public relations and evangelical approaches to dissemination within the organisation, which mirror those most commonly used to publish ideas and developments outside. It has already been argued that such approaches can be counterproductive and are not conducive to effective change management or integration of the PDU into the organisation as a whole, and alternative approaches within the organisation have been discussed in Chapter 4.

To some extent, because of the scale of the exercise, networking outside the confines of one's own usual area of practice will inevitably tend to focus more on exchange of information and ideas, and on discussion of complex or difficult topics, rather than on collaborations targeted on the development of specific practices. However, there can be argued to be merits in each of the approaches, even where there are practical difficulties in their execution, as discussed at the start of this chapter.

Broadly speaking, the PDU has identified four different approaches to networking with professionals from other organisations

Networking by correspondence or telephone

Often this follows publication of PDU work in journals or at conferences. Similarly, the PDU team may identify work of others which is relevant to its own activity. It may also arise from formal lists of network contacts, such as that provided by the King's Fund, or similarly the Centre for the Development of Nursing Policy and Practice networks in Leeds. This is probably the most straightforward form of networking activity and may result simply in the exchange of more detailed information, provision of telephone numbers for further contacts, or discussion of a specific aspect of the published work. Beyond this, however, it may also lead to the arrangement of meetings or visits to discuss issues in more detail.

The PDU as network host

As part of its dissemination strategy, the PDU routinely arranges visits on request for multidisciplinary groups either to examine the development and management of the unit as a whole in more detail, or to discuss a specific practice development. Such visits would routinely include some form of presentation and an opportunity to see the unit in its everyday function, followed by a discussion of issues important to the visitors. While the primary purpose of this activity is dissemination of the unit's work, the team seeks to ensure that, where possible, these events result in a two-way exchange of ideas and information, and where there are issues of mutual interest they may even lead to an ongoing collaboration. An example of this is the unit's collaboration with a hospital near Hull, which is discussed in more detail below.

In this activity, the PDU has played host to visitors from all around the UK, in addition to groups from Europe and the USA. Beyond these routine visits, the unit has regularly hosted seminars and conferences which provide a more formal opportunity for both dissemination of ideas and forming contacts with a wider range of people. In addition, the RAG and Clinical Forum discussed earlier provide vehicles for more *ad hoc* networking where new contacts can be made.

The PDU as network participant

In addition to receiving visitors and hosting events, members of the PDU team also regularly visit other clinical units. This may be to present the PDU approach or work to other teams in their own environment, or for members of the PDU team to learn about specific practices in another organisation. This has been found to be a valuable exercise in exploring the way forward for specific developments. Much can be gleaned prior to instituting a new development from a thorough review of the salient literature. However, only a visit and free discussion with practitioners involved in the development will reveal the real practical complexity of the issues involved and the obstacles which may need to be overcome in implementation. These are areas consistently under-represented in journal articles which naturally focus on results and tend to present work as though it were a logical, uninterrupted progression from theoretical plan to ultimate outcome. This, of course, makes for far more slick published material, but tends not to address the issues which would be of most value to others involved in similar practice developments.

The PDU contributes where possible to seminar and conference presentations and often the most valuable aspect of these events is the opportunity they provide for forming further contacts with colleagues from other organisations. Representatives of the unit also participate regularly in formal network groups established at regional or national level. Such groups tend to meet on a regular basis and to involve named individuals with similar interests or back-grounds from different organisations. Examples of such groups include a nursing Research and Development Group and a Practice Development Group facilitated by the Centre for the Development of Nursing Policy and Practice in Leeds. More recently, an attempt has been made by some interested in the development unit approach to establish a new network of such units.

The value of these formal network groups is in providing time and space for practitioners with shared interests to come together to discuss issues of concern. They facilitate the identification of common priori-ties and the coordination of pressure for change. In addition, they play a strong role in identifying and supporting education and development particularly of the leaders of the networking units by resourcing and supporting developmental programmes. Finally, they have value as vehicles for sharing of information both related to specific practice issues and of a political nature. This last aspect is particularly impor-tant, as political naivety amongst practice developers is a major barrier to success where clinical practice development has to be taken forward in the complex political context of the organisation as a whole.

These benefits have been well described in King's Fund publica-tions about their own NDU network, and are likely to be echoed by any involved in the groups described above. However, there are some limitations to such groups. The first of these is their tendency towards a uni disciplinary focus, which generally arises out of the structure and function of the organisation hosting the network. As organisations develop with a more multidisciplinary remit, it is likely that network groups will be established with a similar breadth of membership. However, the difficulty then will be to retain the interest of practition-ers from very different professional backgrounds and to prevent the domination of the network by one specific professional group.

The second limitation of formal network groups appears to be their poor capacity to engender practical collaborations on specific practice developments. This may relate in part to the way in which such networks operate, or equally to the difficulty of linking together the agendas of different and often competing trusts with very differ-ent and short-term priorities. Whatever the reason, this is a difficult issue for such groups, given the need for practice developers to demonstrate clear concrete outcomes from their activity.

Collaborative developments

The fourth broad approach to networking is that of forging concrete links with other individuals, units or organisations in order to address a specific practice issue. It may be that this approach arises out of the previous forms of networking, although it may equally be possible to start out with the intention of tackling specific problems or ideas. The PDU has sought to focus its networking attentions to a considerable degree on this approach which, as described earlier in the chapter, related the activity of networking most directly to the philosophy of the unit and to its practice development objectives.

Between individual academic and research organisations such collaborations are relatively common. However, between units within health service trusts and other organisations this remains a relatively uncommon phenomenon, and skills in building such links are still developing. The unit's team does not, therefore, claim massive expertise or unfaltering success in this area. Nevertheless, it is a worthwhile exercise to discuss a number of the unit's experiences in order to demonstrate both the potential value of such collaborations and the difficulties which need to be overcome in order to realise this.

The remainder of this chapter will therefore be devoted to an analysis of some of the unit's attempts to pursue this approach to networking; to the perceived benefits of the approach and to its pitfalls. This analysis will focus on four specific collaborations, between the unit and: two trusts in different regions; a trust within the same region; a local university; and a neighbouring NDU.

Collaboration: four examples

Trust network

This network arose out of a collaboration initially between the Chief Nurses of three NHS hospital trusts. From a number of initial discussions emerged the concept of collaborating on several issues of key importance to the trusts. A joint workshop was held involving practice leaders from each trust, and three priority nursing issues were identified:

- care pathways
- research and development
- clinical supervision.

From the workshop, only the issue of clinical supervision emerged as an area where there was potential for collaboration and it was perhaps significant that the representatives from the PDU were involved in this particular sub-group.

Each of the trusts was in the process of developing a pilot approach to clinical supervision and was keen to be able to evaluate its impact on practice. It was agreed that, as each trust was at a different stage of implementing its pilot and as each pilot was different in its details, the collaboration between the trusts would have most benefit if it focused on a common approach to the evaluation of these pilots. The benefits of this would include a pooling of ideas and resources and the ability to compare data, resulting in a more widely applicable and credible study.

Over the following months a number of three-way discussions were arranged in order to take this work forward. The emphasis of the evaluation was on the perceptions, achievements, knowledge and understanding of the individual nurse, rather than on levels of sickness and absence, job satisfaction or other generic measures which were felt likely to be too crude to detect changes in a relatively small pilot exercise. A framework for evaluation was agreed, based on the objectives for clinical supervision set out by one of the network partners. Work then proceeded to design a joint questionnaire based on this framework.

The collaborative exercise encountered difficulties at the outset. These included:

- The different stages of development of the three trusts' pilot exercises. In the first, the pilot was well established, trust-wide and involved the local College of Health. In the PDU's own trust the pilot was small, involving only the unit itself, and at a relatively early stage. In the third trust, the pilot had not yet begun and was only at an early stage of planning.
- The different emphasis placed on the pilot exercises within the three trusts. In the first, the exercise was viewed as a major priority, with considerable resources devoted to it. A substantial structure had been established to support its development. In the PDU's own trust, the development was viewed with some scepticism. The official attitude was one of support in principle for the development and an expressed desire to evaluate closely, but doubt about its cost effectiveness and an apparent preference to see whether it would fly first before it was actively supported. To this extent, the PDU was allowed to run with the project but was not supported in any meaningful sense. Beyond this the PDU had some difficulty itself in accommodating the development, as it related only to one discipline rather than to an issue of multidisciplinary practice and although the potential to examine the issue

in multidisciplinary terms was recognised, this was not felt to be practically feasible within the context of this collaboration. In the third Trust, there appeared to be an imperative to develop some work around clinical supervision, but no priority attached to its development on as broad a scale as the first, nor to its rigorous evaluation.

These issues meant that each trust's representatives attached a different priority to the work in hand, and tended to interpret the objectives of the exercise, although jointly defined, in a subtly different way.

These problems were further exacerbated by the sheer practical difficulty of getting together. Each meeting between the three parties took a minimum of 2–3 months to arrange, and if one party was unable to attend because of a local crisis, as happened on one occasion, this effectively brought the work to a stand still for months.

During the first year of the collaboration, a questionnaire and framework for its implementation were eventually developed. However, the resulting tool was too cumbersome for practical use within the trusts and was in need of further editing and refinement. The scale of the tool was at least in part a reflection of the process of its design – in that designing by committee tended to lead to something which could satisfy all of the participants' different priorities and perspectives.

In the meantime, the pilots had continued to develop internally at different rates and with different levels of success, such that the work of the collaboration no longer appeared to relate equally to the activity in the different trusts and to some extent the opportunity for implementation of the evaluation tool was lost.

Positive outcomes from this activity included a sharing of theoretical knowledge and experiences of implementing clinical supervision which probably benefited most the less advanced trusts. Work on the collaborative evaluation tool continues, between the first trust and PDU only. However, the credibility of this work and hence the resources and effort attached to it have significantly deteriorated with the passage of time with no concrete benefits. The collaboration has also led to a lasting contact and sharing of ideas and information on a broad range of other issues between practitioners in the two teams.

Negative outcomes have included a significant loss of time, energy and other resources on an activity which has yielded little tangible benefit so far for the unit, its patients or staff. The costs in terms of resources and effort have generally outweighed any concrete benefits.

Networking with a trust in the same region

This activity arose out of an initial visit to the PDU by practitioners from the other trust, who had read about the unit's work in journal articles and had met a number of its staff at network groups or conference events. The party came to the PDU to examine its general approach and to gather information about specific developments. This initial visit was successful and was followed by an equally successful reciprocal visit of a party from the PDU to the other trust. Both parties felt that they had learned from the exercise and a number of personal contacts were made and possible areas for future collaboration identified.

One such area was the rehabilitation of patients following a stroke. At this time the Research Practitioner was beginning to develop a number of small projects around stroke care, which had been identified as one of the priorities for development within the unit. As part of this work within the PDU, the Research Practitioner had been attempting to encourage nurses to examine their role in the multidisciplinary approach to stroke rehabilitation and in particular how this interfaced with that of the physiotherapists. Using reflective practice techniques he had facilitated a group of practitioners in evaluation of their own role and performance and had used both published material and critical incidents from the practitioners' own experience to fuel this reflection.

The aim of the exercise was to influence knowledge, attitudes and practice and to evaluate, through the practitioners' own reflections, the extent to which this was being achieved. The work was conceived as a relatively low key experiment in staff development which might merit more rigorous evaluation in due course if early indications proved positive. In addition, it was a method of provoking debate at ward level, encouraging the use of research material in practice and of identifying potential areas for future practice development.

Contacts in the other trust felt that this might also be a useful exercise for their own staff and after initial discussion it was agreed that the Research Practitioner would employ some of his methods with a group from this trust in addition to the group within the PDU. The attractions for the PDU were the additional information this collaboration might provide on the perceptions of nurses of their role in stroke care and on areas for potential development, and the potential for this initial work to lead on to more substantial collaborations in the same area. Initially, the activity appeared to be successful with good attendances by the new group, and the Research Practitioner was hopeful of realising similar benefits with the new group to those which had been apparent within the PDU.

However, after several meetings attendance began to wane, and the reflective activity needed to fuel the discussions was more likely to be forgotten. Ultimately, although the exercise has never been officially abandoned, it has continued to decline steadily.

As with the first example, the reasons for this are probably complex. Firstly, the activity itself is one which is relatively difficult to define, with no obvious specific end-point. Secondly, the exercise was identified as valuable principally by the practice leader in the other trust, rather than by practitioners themselves. Although volunteers came forward to participate, the rationale for the activity may have been less clear to them than to the practitioners in the PDU who had themselves created the impetus for the experiment in discussion with the Research Practitioner. Thirdly, there are many day-to-day practical issues which get in the way of a relatively nebulous exercise like reflection on practice. Within the PDU the Research Practitioner was visible, sometimes working on the wards, always available for discussion and to inquire of individuals' progress. This helped to encourage individuals to use this reflective process and to evaluate their practice. This input from the Research Practitioner was not possible in the partner trust because of his time constraints. Initially, the practice leader and a local tutor undertook this role within the partner trust, but part way through the activity both of these individuals left the organisation and subsequently no new individual champions emerged. A fourth factor related to the PDU itself and its own need some way into the collaboration to refocus its attention within the unit itself in reponse to its own pressures arising from the hospital mergers. For these reasons, reflection and recording of these reflections on practice were increasingly patchy between discussions and although the exercise has continued to be useful within the PDU, its full benefit was never realised through the network collaboration.

Positive outcomes of this activity include continued close contact between the other trust and the PDU and a significant exchange of ideas and information facilitated by the more prolonged contacts and opportunities for discussion. Through this initial collaboration, the Research Practitioner formed a further partnership with a senior academic from the area and a research proposal related to care of stroke patients was submitted. This bid was unfortunately unsuccessful, so that the potential for further concrete collaboration could not be realised at that time.

Negative outcomes were the eventual fading out of the development and the costs of travel and facilitator's time which were at the expense of the PDU and ultimately produced little in the way of tangible developments arising from the external group.

Collaboration with the local university

This collaboration arose out of earlier networking between the two organisations. Early in its establishment the PDU had formed contacts with key staff within the university and had involved them in the planning and support of the unit, via the unit's Steering Group, Clinical Forum and RAG, for example. This close collaboration over many months facilitated the development of many individual contacts and allowed the partners to explore issues of mutual concern in some depth.

Beyond the initial focus on a sharing of skills, knowledge and experience, it was agreed that the essential outcome of this collaboration should be a partnership in development of specific areas of practice of mutual interest. One example of this was a collaboration to investigate the educational needs of newly diagnosed diabetic patients.

This project and its results are discussed in detail in Chapter 9, so we will only comment here on the role of collaboration within this exercise. The project was conceived as one of mutual benefit to the two organisations involved. The PDU wished to examine and develop its practice with regard to diabetic patients. Similarly, there was a desire to engage patients more closely in the unit's developmental work, in line with its patient focused philosophy. Finally, the unit was keen to provide opportunities for development of its staff both in terms of specific clinical knowledge and the ability to apply research-related skills.

The university department wished to develop partnerships with clinical units, in order to 'ground' its educational activities and to promote its clinical research role. To this end it was offering support in time and material resources for certain of its staff, one of whom was the unit's collaborator on this project. The PDU provided the necessary clinical partner, with a shared interest and a positive framework to support collaborative work. The academic collaborator brought with him both an interest in the clinical subject and experience in using focus group techniques to elicit patients' views. In addition, he would be in a position to support the development of any individuals from the PDU involved in the project.

The project, as described in Chapter 9, was developed as a joint exercise throughout and, although progress was slower than anticipated at times because of the difficulty of arranging meetings, successfully achieved its objectives. This initial work involved identifying patients' and their carers' views of their needs for information after diagnosis as diabetic. The next stage in this work is to use this information to inform the development of local information and education provision for newly diagnosed diabetic patients in the future. To this end the collaboration is continuing.

Positive outcomes from this collaboration included development of a rigorous and concrete research study of direct benefit to the unit's patients and of equal interest in the academic sphere. Simultaneously, there was tangible benefit in terms of the development of individuals involved in the project. The success of the work has provided a platform for future collaboration. Ultimately, the additional time and energy needed to coordinate the input to this project from the two organisations were far outweighed by its benefits.

Collaboration between the PDU and a neighbouring NDU

This collaboration was between the PDU and Wards V and W – a King's Fund supported NDU which offered assessment and care for older people with mental health problems. Although on the same hospital site as the PDU, this unit is managed by a different NHS trust, and therefore there are no direct management contacts between the two units. The philosophy of this unit states that they have positive beliefs and values about nursing and health care; and that they believe that by developing their nursing practice they can raise the profile of nursing older people with mental health needs.

In the relatively short history of both the NDU and the PDU, although the PDU emphasis was on multidisciplinary practice, there has existed a culture where nursing support is shared. This has tremendous value in the care of people who may need the nursing 'expertise' of both the units. The initial collaborative work started in response to the way in which patients were transferred between the mental health wards and the medical wards at Seacroft Hospital. These transfers were often initiated by the medical staff in response to patients' changing needs and the perceived demands these placed upon the existing skills and expertise of the nurses.

These transfers between the two units often resulted in:

- poor communication
- poor coordination of care

- professional rivalry and misunderstanding of each other's roles
- dependency on medical staff as decision-makers
- complaints from patients and carers/relatives.

The desires to resolve these problems and to improve the quality of service to patients were therefore major reasons for developing the liaison.

Other objectives were also identified:

- promotion of the professional development of nurses working within the units, developing existing skills to enable nurses to gain a greater understanding of their patients when identifying care needs
- provision of support
- development of the autonomy of the nursing staff.

The liaison work did not set out to avoid transferring patients between the units when their needs became complex, but rather to help nurses identify health needs early on, seek advice and support from practitioners in the specific areas as well as involving their medical colleagues.

Discussion between the units' leaders took place to look at how these objectives could be implemented and, as a result, question-naires were designed and circulated to all nurses working in the two units. The questionnaires illustrated that staff in the two units did indeed communicate with each other, and did often seek advice on a number of practice issues (including, for example: wound care, pres-sure area care/tissue viability, caring for people with dementia, caring for people who hallucinated), but that further development of this networking in day-to-day practice was desirable and could be supported by more focused mechanisms.

Arrangements for exchange of staff from different levels and grades helped consolidate these formal primary nurse links by devel-oping the personal relationships between staff. The partners also set out to promote effective communication and support whilst patients were transferred, by maintaining relationships between the primary nurses helping to coordinate care when and if patients were trans-ferred back to their original ward.

As a result of the survey and the discussions which followed, regu-lar staff exchanges were established and opportunities for joint discussion and development of knowledge and skills in specific areas were organised, wherein practitioners from each team could draw direct benefit from colleagues in the other team.

Positive benefits from this exercise included a far greater mutual understanding of the very different practice issues in the two settings. This helped the two teams to achieve their objectives of improving communication and planning for transfers and understanding of when transfer was needed. In addition, it was of significant benefit to patients who remained on each unit but who exhibited a complex range of both physical and mental health needs. Given that patients rarely fit into our neat organisational boxes, this was not surprisingly quite a common experience. The time commitment for this activity was relatively low, given the close proximity of the partners, and their ability to meet easily and involve significant numbers of staff helped to ensure the success of the development.

Conclusion

It is not possible to reduce the idea of networking to one simple activity, with clearly defined aims and easily measured outcomes. As discussed above, the word 'networking' is an umbrella term which covers a multitude of sins – from jetting around the continent to various cheese and wine parties, to finding and collaborating with specific partners to develop concrete work of mutual interest.

The unit believes that there is benefit to be gained from all types of networking activity and the PDU approach is, therefore, pragmatic and multifaceted. However, the activity can be perceived as an extremely nebulous phenomenon, the benefits of which are only for an elite few and do not justify the resources applied to it. This is a particularly dangerous perception for a development unit, where a lack of focus to networking may only serve to fuel existing preconceptions and prejudices concerning elitism. With these issues in mind, the PDU has developed a broad general approach to networking, but one which concentrates its resources and energy on activity which reflects the philosophy of the unit and explicitly furthers its concrete development objectives. This form of networking activity brings with it the most tangible benefits within the unit, and also employs available resources most judiciously for the benefit of both the unit itself and for others involved in the network. Its outcomes are also the most easily measured.

Nevertheless, this approach is not without its difficulties and pitfalls, as is evident from the examples given earlier in this chapter. By its very nature it is more complex than activity undertaken within the unit. The challenge, then, is to achieve the potential benefits of such an approach, while minimising the great potential for failure arising from its complexity. As a result of the team's experiences in this area, ten criteria have been identified which are likely to determine the success or otherwise of a specific collaborative networking exercise. They are as follows:

- **Proximity of partners:** The closer one's partner geographically, the easier it is to get together to plan and implement developments collaboratively. The greater the distance, the more expensive and time-consuming the activity tends to become, and the slower the progress and greater the likelihood of unforeseen delays.

  Clearly, wider access to new communication technology will tend to reduce this effect. However, given the intensely practical nature of practice development activity and the need to address the multitude of nitty-gritty issues in practice to achieve change, there remains no real substitute for face-to-face detailed discussion to tease out important issues.

- **Small number of partners:** It is probably self-evident that the more individuals or groups in a network, the greater the potential benefits of sharing information and ideas, and of collaborative work. However, the larger the network, the greater also is the potential for failure. Networks with multiple partners, particularly those at some distance, are particularly time-consuming, expensive and difficult to coordinate. In addition, there is greater risk of incompatibility of philosophies and objectives. Units using a collaboration to support specific practical developments should aim to keep the partnership as small as possible. To achieve success in practical collaborations between multiple partners requires a clear and enduring commitment from all host organisations and a sound resource-base, in addition to all of the other factors described here.

- **Discrete issue for development:** Complex, multifaceted issues form useful subject matter for networks aimed at raising debate, sharing ideas or information. However, if practical development is the aim, then, given the complexity of networking and collaborative project work arrangements, in order to achieve concrete developments it is essential that the chosen area of development is relatively discrete, easily defined and measurable.

- **Partners with a shared interest:** Partners – either individuals or an organisation – who share one's interest in the specific practice issue. Where the partner is an organisation, identification of one or more key individuals remains essential in order to ensure that the issue is driven forward and supported in all areas.

- **Partners with a similar philosophy:** When developing work collaboratively, it is important that the partners are able to 'speak the same language' in terms of their approach to developmental work. If one partner fundamentally believes in a top-down, big bang approach, for example, while another believes in a bottom-up and staged approach, it is unlikely they will be able to arrive at a mutually acceptable change strategy. This is a relatively crude example, but other issues which could influence success might include the extent of any multidisciplinary ethos, receptiveness of staff to change, value placed on the activity by managers, or considerations of relative status (for example, large teaching hospital over relatively small district general hospital).

- **Complementary knowledge, experience and skills:** It is helpful to collaborate with partners who possess knowledge, experience and skills which complement one's own. In this way, the maximum breadth of perspective can be brought to bear on the subject. Good examples of this are the PDU's collaboration with the mental health unit. Others might include a partnership between service and academia, between clinical practitioners of different disciplines, or between individuals in similar organisations where the subject itself is so vast that it is difficult for one individual or group to encompass it.

- **Partners at a similar stage of development:** Even where there is a shared interest in a specific issue, there is likely to be a greater chance of success in collaborative work where all partners enter the activity at a similar level. It is important that all partners are able to start the planned development from a similar baseline to ensure smooth project planning. If experiences and understanding are comparable, this also helps to ensure that all are equal participants is any debates and that no one party feels either swept along at too fast a pace, or that they are carrying an unfair proportion of the burden.

- **Clearly defined and compatible objectives:** It is essential that the objectives of any collaborative exercise are clearly defined and communicated at the outset. This is important for all network partners and for the staff involved. In this way, the partners can demonstrate the value of the activity to their overall aims, can justify the resources used in its implementation, and can build support for the work both inside and outside their unit or department. In addition, clearer objectives at the outset will help to facilitate a more concrete evaluation of the activity.

- **Supporting frameworks in each area:** Each partner in the collaboration needs to have in place frameworks and systems which will support the planning and implementation of the desired development. If this is not the case, there is a danger that work will progress more effectively in one area than in another.
- **'Ownership' in all areas:** Measures need to be taken in all areas involved with a collaborative exercise to develop a sense of ownership of the development among staff. It is possible for a project to be 'worked up' in one place and then, as a result of a network, to co-opt a second organisation into the project. This can result in relatively early success in implementation. However, there are also dangers in this approach, where the staff of the second unit are interested but not fully engaged in the development and where this is seen to be owned by someone from outside the organisation rather than by themselves.

An attempt has been made to describe and analyse some of the practical issues in effective networking, as well as its pitfalls and the benefits which can be achieved if these are overcome. The ten criteria above have been offered as a tool to aid the planning of effective networks focused on practical collaboration.

Networking has been one of the keys to the success of the PDU since its inception. The skills of the PDU team in this area are continuing to develop, but past experiences and failures have enabled them to define far more clearly their expectations of any networking or collaborative activity and their role within it. In an area so complex, resource intensive and fraught with potential pitfalls, the dangers for a development unit are immense. In order to realise the considerable benefits without falling prey to these dangers, this clarity is all-important.

Chapter 11
Dissemination of Practice Development Unit work

Steve Page

The dissemination of its work is integral to the activity of the PDU, not just a 'bolt-on' extra. Because of this, many elements of the PDU approach to dissemination have already been previously discussed in other parts of the book – in particular Chapter 10 on the subject of networking and Chapter 4 which focused on the integration of the unit with, and maximising its benefits to, the wider organisation.

These sections related mainly to the potential of the PDU for driving change within its own organisation or beyond. It is not proposed here to repeat the issues discussed in these earlier chapters. Rather, the intention of this chapter is to take a detailed look at some of the more basic approaches to dissemination as a means of sharing information and ideas to support change – the bread and butter of dissemination activity which underpins and complements the more sophisticated change strategies.

The chapter begins with an overview of how the PDU's approach to dissemination as a whole has evolved, and then outlines a number of distinct aims of internal and external dissemination. The remainder of the chapter then focuses on the diverse approaches adopted by the unit to basic dissemination of its work, seeking to draw out the pros and cons of each different approach in order, hopefully, to aid practitioners in other units to plan their own dissemination strategy.

Evolution of the PDU approach

In one of its early documents, the purpose of the PDU as defined by its original team was summarised as follows:

213

- to serve as a laboratory for innovations in practice and patient care
- to produce and publish research
- to disseminate innovations in order to support the development of patient care
- to act as a demonstration centre for new developments
- to be a resource for the whole organisation.

Clearly, even at this early stage, a heavy emphasis was placed on the need to share work undertaken in the PDU in order to benefit patient care beyond the confines of the unit itself. This emphasis has remained unaltered over time, although the approaches adopted by the unit have continued to evolve. Early in its development, the focus of the PDU's resources tended to be internal, in order to establish its own culture and identity and to support concrete developments in practice within the unit itself. Initial efforts were dedicated to engaging the unit's own staff in this process, as well as to 'selling' the unit to the organisation's managers.

Once the PDU was sufficiently well established and a number of successful developments began to emerge, the unit was able gradually to shift its focus to outside its own confines. Initial audiences for PDU work were principally staff working in other areas within the hospital and nursing colleagues from around the region, facilitated by the Yorkshire region's nursing department. To a great extent this activity was about simple sharing of information and ideas – about specific development work such as self-medication and multidisciplinary record keeping, and soon also about the PDU concept itself.

At this stage, prior to the restructuring of the regional health authority, its nursing network was very active and there was a considerable 'buzz' around the region. The PDU shared its work, along with many others, in an atmosphere which encouraged receptiveness to ideas. In addition, the dissemination of its work was of crucial importance to the unit, both as a celebration of its achievements which would motivate the team, and as a means of demonstrating its value to the hospital's managers.

As the unit continued to evolve, it began to outgrow its regional and unidisciplinary stage and the potential became apparent to share the unit's work with a far broader audience. With this in mind, the unit began to publish its first papers and from these the steady stream of contacts and visits from other organisations across the country began. Initially, papers were published in nursing journals, although authors included members of other disciplines. Gradually, however, this has changed, so that PDU work has now been published in a wide variety of journals – nursing, medical, therapy and management – and at conferences representing the full range of disciplines. This has brought with it a broadening of the unit's range of contacts and visits.

Internally, the unit developed its multidisciplinary records system and subsequently implemented this across the hospital in all specialities. In addition, the Clinical Leader of the unit was developing an increasing involvement in hospital-wide teaching programmes and gradually others from a variety of disciplines were being drawn into this process.

As the hospital organisation evolved, so the PDU involvement also developed. The Leader became an integral part of the organisation's Clinical Practice Group, influencing wider developments in other areas through this forum. From this approach a strategy for internal dissemination gradually emerged which reflected more closely the team's understanding of how change in practice works. The marketing of finished PDU ideas to other areas diminished as the team began to understand how this tended to fuel the perception of the unit as elitist and consequently also to result in a profound resistance to change initiated by it. In its place the unit sought to develop a more collaborative approach, where the PDU was one partner in a developmental venture, able to offer specific qualities to support the change.

This has continued to develop within the unit itself, and now forms the bedrock of its approach to internal dissemination, with the information-sharing mechanism used only as a means to support this activity. The current approach now clearly distinguishes between external dissemination, which is primarily about ideas and information, and internal dissemination, principally about supporting a change in practice on the ground. Externally, the PDU seeks to provide material which will demonstrate the potential value or otherwise of a given approach to care, and ideas which will stimulate multidisciplinary debate and development. Internally, in addition to these effects, the unit aims both to support the development and implementation of innovative multidisciplinary practices which are relevant to all areas involved and, perhaps more importantly, to influence the development of a culture in other parts of the organisation which will support such innovation. This is a far cry from the simple distribution of information and demands a significantly greater effort and risk on the part of the unit. However, the potential for the unit to fulfil its purpose as an engine for change is also proportionately greater.

Aims of dissemination

Superficially, the aims of any dissemination are clear – simply to share information about one's own good ideas or practices with others in order to help them to realise similar benefits in their own areas. In fact, there is somewhat more to the activity than this. As already noted, target audiences for dissemination may differ widely. For example, the target audience may all be from within the same discipline or may be multidisciplinary. It may be within the host organisation or from further afield; its practice specialism may be identical or very different. The aims of dissemination may be similarly multifaceted and may differ in emphasis depending on the specific audience to be addressed.

These aims may include:

- Provision of results of specific project work or developments in order to stimulate similar developments in other areas, or to persuade others of the value or otherwise of developing a similar practice.
- Provision of information about implementation of specific developments, in order, as above, to help stimulate similar developments elsewhere and also to help others to plan a subsequent implementation which avoids similar pitfalls.
- Sharing of ideas to stimulate broader multidisciplinary debate and encourage consideration of innovative approaches in different areas.
- Celebration of achievements in order to reward and motivate the team which has undertaken the work.
- Promotion of the unit in order to gain recognition or support either from inside the host organisation or beyond, or to promote recruitment of new staff.
- Sharing the concept and approach of the PDU itself in order to help others to develop similar units within their own practice areas.
- Sharing the PDU's ideas and resources with other areas in order to actively support the implementation and acceptance of specific change.
- Influencing the culture of other areas through direct contact in order to promote a similar ethos and approach to multidisciplinary innovation, although not necessarily using the PDU structure.

The aims outlined above could all be argued to apply at times to any dissemination activity whether targeted internally to the PDU itself or its host organisation, or externally, and it is clear that these aims are far from being mutually exclusive. However, the last two of these aims, while not entirely irrelevant to activity outside the unit itself or its host organisation are less likely to be achieved on this scale than within the unit's own organisation, where they are the basis of the PDU's internal strategy for dissemination. These have been discussed amply in earlier chapters and therefore it is proposed here to concentrate on techniques to provide information and ideas to support innovation, which are the basis of the unit's external dissemination approaches, as well as being an essential underpinning for the more sophisticated change-oriented approaches.

The PDU as provider of information and ideas to support change

The PDU profile

Since its first year, the PDU has produced a profile which outlines its philosophy and aims and describes its constituent parts and supporting mechanisms. This is a valuable tool for inducting new staff and students and is used widely in helping others to appreciate the differences between the unit and other clinical settings. Hundreds of copies have been distributed widely to professionals from other organisations across the country and abroad, with an interest in developing a similar unit.

Reports on PDU projects

The unit attempts always to produce a written report summarising the implementation and results of any developmental work. This is important as it enables future work to build steadily on previous efforts, rather than having continually to go back over old ground. These reports provide valuable source material to share with other practitioners both internally and externally, and have also been circulated in large numbers. These internal reports can deal in more detail with the processes of implementation than is commonly possible in externally published work which tends to deal more with 'results' and 'successes'. Lessons learned about implementation in a multidisciplinary setting – successful or otherwise – are a key part of the PDU's value to others. In addition to these benefits, the internal reports provide a mechanism to help evaluate the achievements of the unit over a period of time. Latterly, all reports published internally by the PDU have been presented in a 'corporate style' which is aimed at helping to promote the concept of the unit and also to foster the feeling of achievement in those working within it.

Internal exhibitions

These are used within the PDU to ensure its own staff are well informed and may take the form of dedicated noticeboards or mobile exhibition boards. They are also employed elsewhere in the busy areas of the hospitals, in order to raise awareness of specific ideas or developments. They are often used as one part of a strategy for implementation of a specific change.

Teamwork – the PDU Newsletter

The newsletter is published every two months and circulated widely within the PDU and across the trust hospitals, as well as externally in response to inquiries. This newsletter presents an informal summary of current activity which is easily digestible. It promotes the celebration of achievements and is a vehicle for acknowledging the input of individuals to PDU successes. It provides valuable contacts within the PDU for those wishing to pursue an issue further and, finally, helps to reinforce the PDU identity.

Presentations to hospital/trust groups

A number of audit, research and practice development forums exist across the trust and these are frequently used as a vehicle for presenting PDU work. The advantage of such forums is that they tend to be organised already and to draw from various areas across the organisation, so that their use entails relatively little effort in reaching a reasonably broad audience. On the negative side, these groups tend to be unidisciplinary or at least dominated by one discipline, so that the PDU message can be hard to convey in a simple presentation or may only be perceived to be partly relevant to a unidisciplinary audience. Positive outcomes from the use of such forums in the hospital have been principally through the use of the clinical audit meetings. Regularly presenting PDU work in these meetings has promoted the development of a strong multidisciplinary focus in audit work in place of the previously medically dominated forum. Tying in the audit activity explicitly to the work of the PDU's Clinical Forum has facilitated the completion of the audit cycle by providing a mechanism to take forward actions arising from audit work, or supplying ideas from practice which might merit audit work.

The PDU Clinical Forum

This weekly multidisciplinary meeting provides an opportunity for practitioners to share ideas for future work or discuss progress or results of current projects. It is also a mechanism for simple sharing of information between team members, and is valuable in continuing to support the PDU's team and in maintaining its identity as a unit. The Clinical Forum has, in addition, proved to be a valuable mechanism for more active support of internal dissemination. Its linkage with clinical audit and uses as a driver of change have also been described in detail in Chapter 4.

Journal papers

Papers are a useful mechanism for dissemination, both internally and externally. To start with, the target was mainly nursing publications, but more recently the PDU has published in a wide range of clinical and managerial journals. This has helped to broaden the audience for the unit's message and to further promote the multidisciplinary approach to care, as well as any specific aspect of clinical practice.

It can be difficult involving clinical staff in such activity, as many lack writing skills or, more often, simply the confidence to write. The PDU has put considerable effort into supporting the broader involvement of staff in this activity, and routine production of internal reports has been a valuable mechanism to facilitate this.

Although journals exist in absurd numbers and questions are asked about their capacity to really influence practice, they have been found within the PDU to be an effective means of disseminating ideas and generating further interest. The publication of each successive journal article has fuelled an increasing number of telephone and postal enquiries, and visits to the unit to discuss either how to set up and run such a unit or the PDU's approach to developing a specific aspect of practice.

In addition, as with internal reports, such publications can be used (with caution) as a means of evaluating the unit's performance. They also raise the credibility of the unit – to clinical professions who particularly value scientific publications, to academics and to managers. Finally, they are a significant means of celebrating achievements and rewarding effort.

External seminars

Various members of the PDU team have presented work at external seminars. These have included groups of pre-registration students and various network groups. As with presentations to established groups within the organisation, one disadvantage of this approach is that the audiences tend to be composed predominantly of practitioners from one discipline only, so that the PDU message is slightly harder to convey. A further disadvantage, particularly with network groups, is that they tend to be composed of a relatively small number of people who share specific interests. While this is in some respects advantageous, in others there may sometimes be an element of 'preaching to the converted'.

External seminars are, however, useful in that they provide a relatively informal and focused setting, in which the nuances of PDU work can be discussed in detail and grey areas clarified. They are therefore effective in stimulating critical thinking about multidisciplinary development and often lead to further contacts and possibly also to practical collaboration. In addition, such seminars have been found to be a useful mechanism to promote recruitment to the unit of staff with a similar philosophy and dissatisfaction with the status quo.

Conferences/exhibitions

Members of the PDU team have presented papers and exhibits at a wide range of regional and national events. Such events have proven a useful way of stimulating further contacts from interested practitioners. They are a means of disseminating the PDU message to a wider and possibly more diverse audience. Other benefits obviously include increasing the reputation and credibility of the unit in key quarters, and the boost this activity offers to the morale of staff working in the unit and in particular those involved in the specific developments presented.

On the negative side, however, the nature of large conferences and exhibitions is such that there is scant opportunity to go into detail about PDU work. Presentations tend to be superficial 'flavours' of any given subject rather than in-depth analyses, and the crucial message of the unit can easily be lost in the diversity of presentations. Often, at a large event, only a proportion of the programme is of interest to each delegate and therefore the message can be still harder to convey. The annual round of conferences and exhibitions has proliferated enormously over recent years and has become something of an industry, such that the value of many events to clinical practice can be questionable. Participation in such events by a small unit needs to be carefully managed to achieve maximum benefit, since it can be both a time-consuming and, if one is not part of the relative minority of national figures in the paid lecture circuit, also quite an expensive pursuit.

Annual PDU conference/exhibition

Each year the PDU has sought to host its own event. This has generally taken the form of a combination of small conference, discussion and demonstration workshops, exhibition and tours around the unit with members of the team. These events have been a useful means of dissemination, in that the programme of events is entirely defined by the unit and the audience multidisciplinary, reflecting the promotion of the event. This provides an opportunity to discuss issues in detail and to respond to specific practical queries from enthusiasts and sceptics alike. It allows interested people to hear about and discuss the theoretical aspects of the unit and its work and to see how this theory is applied first hand as they visit the unit. In addition, it allows a rare opportunity for debate and exchange of ideas across disciplines.

Planning for such an event stimulates a considerable amount of discussion within the unit and makes the team critically re-examine each time what they are about, why the PDU is different to other units, and what key message they wish to convey. The event is therefore a valuable tool to promote critical thinking and team cohesion within the unit.

In addition, of course, the events have proven extremely valuable as a means of raising the profile and status of the PDU itself, both externally and within its own organisation. The importance of the latter, as discussed in earlier chapters, cannot be overestimated in terms of the continued survival of a small unit in the current high-pressure NHS climate.

Finally, these events are a very effective means of celebrating the unit's achievements and of promoting its identity internally. They allow opportunity for a broad cross-section of the team to participate and are both a significant reward for hard work on PDU developments and a means of developing new skills and experience in staff who are relatively unused to presenting work to others.

The only negative issue in this approach is the intense effort and amount of time and other resources required to mount the events. Rarely is there additional administrative support available, so that the organisation takes place in addition to any existing activity, and the work involved in organising even a small conference and exhibition can be considerable. As noted elsewhere, although they can produce all of the benefits listed above and, if managed properly, can even help to boost the PDU's funds, there is a significant risk involved in diverting valuable time and effort away from actual development within the unit. It should not be forgotten, either, that there is always the potential for them to fail to attract an audience and therefore both to make a financial loss and to have the opposite to all of the other desired effects. With this in mind, such events may work best for units which are already relatively well-known, and while the PDU has itself had only positive experiences with this approach, the events have certainly attracted a more substantial and varied audience and been more successful, as the unit and its work have become more widely known.

Ad hoc educational sessions

Like many clinical departments, the unit frequently organises and delivers semi-formal teaching sessions for groups of staff both within the unit and in the broader organisation. These most frequently relate to new developments and are usually a part of a broader strategy for implementation of a new practice. As well as being a useful means of supporting new developments, they are also valuable internally for inducting new staff into the unit. Wherever possible, the sessions are delivered by different members of the PDU multidisciplinary team involved in the specific developments, and the target audiences are also multidisciplinary. This helps to reinforce the PDU message. In addition, these sessions can be clearly demonstrated to relate to organisational priorities and to tie in to other areas of work across the organisation. Such sessions also provide opportunities for staff from a range of disciplines to work together and present material in a relatively non-threatening environment, and to develop their own skills in the process.

Formal education programmes

The organisation of which the PDU is part has a formal education and training programme. The content of this programme is determined by a form of annual needs analysis as well as by organisation-level priorities. The PDU has consistently made a substantial contribution to this programme. This has taken the form of sessions on clinical priorities led by PDU staff seen to be leading practice in those areas – for example: nutritional assessment, multidisciplinary assessment, discharge planning, and moving and handling. In addition, PDU leaders have contributed sessions to trust staff on broader areas related to the unit's work such as supporting innovation and change in practice, the appreciation and application of research, quality improvement, and legal and professional issues in record keeping.

This linkage of the PDU work and approaches into formal trust education and training programmes enables the unit to clearly demonstrate its value to the organisation. It also facilitates the transmission of the PDU message to others without the appearance of evangelism, since this message itself is implicit in the aims and content of the session rather than explicit.

Places on these formal programmes are often sold to practitioners from outside the trust and this is therefore another means of disseminating information to audiences not necessarily reached by other means, such as nursing home staff, practice nurses or other multidisciplinary professionals working for social services.

Beyond this, members of the PDU team have written diploma modules for a local university, based on the unit's work, as well as contributing to other taught courses outside. Two of the PDU staff were also invited to write and deliver a module for a nursing master's degree course, in which examples of practice from the PDU and issues of inter-disciplinary collaboration were introduced to stimulate debate.

Such formal educational opportunities enable the unit to reach different groups of practitioners. They help to provide external endorsement for the value of the unit's work. In addition, they enable the unit's ideas to be introduced – particularly at master's level – in a forum in which they can be critically analysed and debated alongside other approaches to practice and its development. This is valuable both to students and to the unit's team in reflection on their own ideas and practice.

Involvement in formal educational programmes, therefore, has considerable benefits, and may also earn funds to support the unit's work. However, they can entail a significant time commitment and with success this tends to increase with new invitations. This can be seductive in terms of the visible achievement associated with them, but needs to be balanced carefully against the primary function of the PDU – of developing and evaluating practice.

Presentations to other development units

On occasions, members of the PDU team have visited other units in early stages of development, in order to address that unit's steering group or other key individuals. This has been relatively infrequent and has tended to be focused on issues of philosophy, organisation and practical support, rather than on specific clinical developments

– the purpose of the exercise being to share experiences and help define some of the pitfalls and ways to avoid these, and also to convince selected individuals whose support is essential, of the merits of the approach. This tends to be a difficult and abstract exercise without tangible examples of the PDU's work to illustrate the theory. However, it may be the only exposure that senior consultants and managers in an organisation get to such ideas from outside their organisation, and therefore may be an important form of endorsement for clinical staff involved. The extent to which this is the case has been difficult to gauge.

Telephone contacts

These are frequent (for example, around 30 during the last six months of 1995) from practitioners in other organisations and may relate to specific areas of practice or to the PDU itself, where others wish to embark on a similar venture. They tend to follow conference or seminar presentations or publication of articles, and are responded to initially by the PDU Leader or Research Practitioner. Usually material such as internal reports or Profiles are sent out in the post and not uncommonly they lead on to further telephone discussions with appropriate members of the unit team or to subsequent visits by inquiring practitioners.

Visits to the PDU

Following initial contact through many of the sources described above, many groups of practitioners have asked to visit the PDU. In the last six months of 1995, for example, 41 visitors were received from 14 different organisations.

These visits have tended to take the form of presentations about the PDU and any subjects of specific interest to the visitors, followed by an opportunity for discussion with PDU staff who have worked on these subjects, and ultimately a tour around the unit. The basic presentation tends to be made by the PDU Leader and Research Practitioner, with other members of the clinical team co-opted as appropriate. This might include members of the multidisciplinary team leading a specific project or might simply reflect the composition of the visiting team. For example, where visitors interested in developing a PDU include an occupational therapist or physiotherapist, they not unnaturally wish to meet their opposite numbers in order to hear at first hand the implications, practical issues and benefits for their profession of the PDU approach.

The benefits of hosting visits to the PDU as a method of dissemination are considerable. They enable the message to be tailored to visitors' needs and allow time for in-depth discussion. Ideas from other areas can be shared with the unit's team and often further contact ensues related to areas of mutual interest. Furthermore, the visits can be a morale boost to the unit's staff who can see that they are a part of something 'special', and they are a very effective means of involving a broader cross-section of the team and of developing skills.

The visits are, however, extremely time-consuming – approximately half a day for each, in addition to the preparatory work. They are labour intensive and in particular require the input of staff with clinical case-loads. They can, therefore, be difficult to maintain in a relatively small unit like the PDU. As the unit has become more experienced in handling them, visits have tended to be grouped at intervals, rather than dealing with each organisation separately. This bringing together of practitioners from different organisations has also had knock-on benefits in terms of enriching the discussions. In addition, a portfolio of standard materials has been prepared and refined for presentation on the range of subjects of interest to visitors, so that the presentation can be tailored to individual needs with a minimum of work by selecting materials from this portfolio.

Finally, a small fee for visitors has been introduced, as well as for materials sent out by post. This is partly to cover costs because of the increasing expense of responding to external enquiries, but also to ensure that visits and requests for information are from genuinely interested parties. At one point it became almost impossible to keep up with information requests as they tended to be undifferentiated and simply to ask for 'one of everything' – rather like the frenzy of freebie-collecting that takes hold of some practitioners at professional exhibitions.

These measures have enabled the team to manage the process more effectively, to give a better quality of experience to visitors and to maintain a more effective balance between the demands of hosting such visits and of clinical practice and development.

Visits from abroad

The PDU has hosted visits from several groups of nurses from France as well as staff from a range of professional groups from the USA and several other European countries. An exchange agreement was forged between the hospital and a partner in Lille, based largely around the PDU. While several visits were hosted, only one party was able to make the return trip to France, owing to lack of available funds to support the venture. Given the significant differences in health care organisation and practice even around Europe, debate between practitioners from different countries is potentially very valuable. This is beginning to be recognised, and it is important that this recognition is accompanied by provision of resources to support clinical-level contact and debate as well as that by purely academic institutions.

Information technology

The PDU has made very effective use of computer technology in its basic activities – for example, data analysis, report writing and production of publicity materials. However, dissemination on a national or international level is potentially facilitated by access to recent developments in information technology, such as e-mail and the Internet. To date, the PDU has not been able to avail itself of this technology, other than through university libraries or by contributing to existing project databases. However, there is undoubtedly considerable scope to explore these avenues in the future.

In academic circles this technology is now readily available and access is beginning to increase in practice settings via clinical audit and R&D departments. Effective networks between the PDU and these departments are therefore increasingly vital. However, these remain one step removed from clinical practice itself, and the essential next step in bringing such information technology to bear more directly on clinical practice development is to bring the resource directly into clinical units. This would enable the unit to access research evidence to underpin its developments as well as a wide variety of other multidisciplinary information. It would facilitate networking between units, and between clinical practitioners and educationalists – vastly speeding up collaborative work. In addition, it would provide a further means of dissemination of ideas and information to a potentially vast audience.

The number of practitioners who are capable of using such information technology is growing and is likely to be relatively high in a unit whose ethos promotes development and innovation. Nevertheless, as well as the resource gap in terms of equipment provision, there remains a considerable information technology skills gap which needs to be addressed urgently, if clinical practitioners are to make maximum use of the available technology.

Conclusion

An essential component of the PDU, as identified in Chapter 2, is the dissemination of its work to others. This can operate on the relatively simple level of provision of information or ideas to stimulate debate or to support a change in practice, or on the more complex level of actively driving change in other areas through the PDU's various mechanisms. Throughout this book, the intention has been to demonstrate how this activity is integral to the function of the unit as a whole, rather than being viewed as an optional extra activity.

In this chapter, the range of methods developed and employed by the unit for the sharing of information and ideas has been discussed in some detail. The unit's team believe these activities to be of value in themselves, as well as being an essential underpinning for the more sophisticated change strategies.

The PDU's approach to dissemination of information and ideas has been developed largely through a process of trial and error – through reflection on what appears to have worked and what does not, on what 'feels right'. This has led the unit to develop a view of the various dissemination techniques as something similar to items in a tool-kit which can be used either individually or in combination, in order to tackle a specific job. Different tasks will require different tools for their completion, and the more complex the task, the greater the combination of tools which will be required. As the unit has developed, so the understanding of its leaders of the range of tools available and of their relative merits and pitfalls has increased. The value of this is that it has enabled a more strategic approach to the planning of dissemination for any given issue and has also increasingly helped to minimise any wastage of time and resources, which can be considerable.

There is clear evidence from within its own hospital of the impact of PDU dissemination on specific practices as well as on the culture in general. The unit's current challenge in this respect within its new organisation is dauntingly large, and yet there still appears to be a recognition that the unit and its team have influenced Trust-wide thinking about multidisciplinary practice, and may be able to exert further influence through the developing clinical effectiveness agenda. In addition, there has been much informal feedback from other organisations and individuals to indicate the extent to which the PDU's ideas and input have been valued. However, one of the great regrets of the PDU team is that no formal evaluation of the impact of its dissemination outside its own organisation has so far been undertaken. The team is well aware of the breadth of its external dissemination activity, having maintained records in recent years of the numbers and sources of individual inquiries and visits, its publications and other public presentations, including citation in others' work and latterly its inclusion in a BBC video package (BBC, 1995). However, it has not collected feedback from its contacts on the specific influence of the PDU's ideas and information within their own areas.

In conclusion then, there are three key points which any unit would do well to consider when planning widespread dissemination of its work. The first is to ensure that dissemination activity is planned as part of the work of the unit as a whole and is considered as an integral part of any specific project planning. The second is to define the objectives of any dissemination at the outset, to consider carefully the range of techniques available and to employ these in a planned and coordinated manner which reflects these objectives, the audience to be targeted, the subject matter to be shared and the resources available. The final key point is the need to evaluate the impact of dissemination activity both as a means of informing future planning in this area and of demonstrating the value of the unit as a positive influence for change.

Chapter 12
The contribution of
the Seacroft PDU

Sally Casley, David Allsopp, Steve Page and Angela Turner

This chapter attempts to review the progress and contribution of the PDU, using as its basis the six essential components of the 'model' which have remained constant throughout its six-year history. Its development and achievements will be considered in the context of continued organisational change. The discussion also reviews the PDU as part of the continued national growth of development units and the refinement of approaches to their accreditation. Finally, the chapter considers the future potential of the PDU approach.

For the Seacroft unit a different path has been necessary in response to changing circumstances. However, to some extent the PDU approach, its principles and ways of working, are only now coming into their own, whether used as a single, coherent model or adapted to inform practice in existing settings. The approach of the unit will be argued to relate directly to current health service debates: on clinical effectiveness and the multi-factorial nature of implementing clinical guidelines, on considerations of quality and efficiency in complex healthcare processes, and on the need to consider healthcare delivery and organisation in ways which cross traditional organisational boundaries.

Staff empowerment

The PDU was established in part to facilitate the bringing together of two hospitals so that they could function effectively as one, recognising that the key to success would be the development of staff from both sites into one effective team. In the earliest days at St George's

Hospital it was the need to develop the staff to cope with a more acute medical workload which drove things forward. Key elements of the approach adopted by the hospitals' managers at this time revolved around the empowerment of the workforce – through the development of new skills and knowledge, through facilitation of multidisciplinary team-working (building on existing strengths), and through the creation of new opportunities for participation in debates and decision making about the future shape and management of their service. These new approaches helped bring about the successful amalgamation of the two hospitals and the creation of a new, positively charged unit, where critical reflection on practice and debates about new ways of working were increasingly the norm.

One of the features of NHS culture which can inhibit innovation in practice is the way in which power is distributed through a hierarchical and rigidly demarcated structure of hospital organisation. Not only do we see hierarchies within professions, but between them too. Medicine has a historical place at the 'top' of the tree and others are traditionally placed in debatable order 'beneath' them. At the same time, nursing, therapies, pharmacy, management and so on, can be established as entirely separate departments, with divergent roles and measures of success. Whilst such hierarchies and structures can provide mechanisms for accountability and effective operation within individual departments, innovation in practice and effective patient care across the service are more difficult within such a rigid framework.

Within the emerging PDU a culture was created which broke down some of these hierarchies and rigid demarcations, encouraging the participation of staff at all grades, facilitating the devolution of decision making to a level closer to the patient, and enabling the critical review and development of processes of care across departmental boundaries.

Management forum meetings were created where everyone was welcome. Business planning issues were openly discussed and staff were free to contribute to discussions in ways which were quite exceptional for the NHS. The management style of the Clinical Director and Service Manager was one of openness, with a real commitment to multidisciplinary working and involvement at all levels.

In addition, a considerable emphasis was also placed on the development of management skills and responsibility among the ward sisters and departmental heads, to support decision making closer to the ground. This was mirrored also in the development of primary nursing within the wards, which in itself increased the autonomy of staff within the ward teams. These developments created a situation where new ideas and innovations could readily be identified and taken up, without the need for checking and permission via cumbersome administrative systems.

These basic changes in the management and organisation of the unit were further supported over time by the development of multidisciplinary clinical groups, which also facilitated the involvement of staff in open debates about practice.

A variety of management and clinical forums were therefore created where those working on the unit could develop a shared philosophy and set of goals, which greatly enhanced the ability of the unit to drive forward changes in practice. Similarly, the explicit links between management and clinical practice, between business and practice development goals, have been important features of the PDU's success by reducing friction between the two agendas and ensuring that the work of the whole team is aimed broadly in the same direction. Over time, the PDU has successfully adapted its structures and approaches to work in order to continue to achieve these basic goals.

A considerable emphasis was placed within the PDU on the development of skills and knowledge of individual staff. This was not merely through the use of formal courses and study days. In addition to these more formal methods, emphasis was given to personal development through multidisciplinary project work, networking, shadowing of skilled practitioners and other more tailored approaches, which were related back to the goals of the unit via PDU action planning and the Individual Personal Review (IPR) process.

The unit's success in this area was reflected in its selection by the Trust as a pilot site for work towards the Investors in People standard. The focus of this standard on the development of individuals as a means of achieving the business goals of the organisation, the linkage of the process of individual personal development to these goals, and the emphasis on structured evaluation of progress, were seen to be very much in keeping with the philosophy and approach of the PDU.

Such approaches have reaped dividends within the unit, and in addition to ensuring a steady stream of practice development activity of a high calibre, have also been a significant factor in recruitment and retention of staff. Similarly, the benefits to individuals of the PDU approach have been readily demonstrated in the career progressions of those leaving the unit. In a recent survey of staff views of the PDU

(Allsopp and Page, 1995) it was noted by respondents that working on the PDU was quite different to working anywhere else. The PDU was felt by most to have provided opportunities not usually found elsewhere. Around half those surveyed felt they could make a real contribution to developing practice in the PDU. Many said they were actively encouraged to suggest new approaches on their wards, and to question practice and try out new ideas.

Such developments have not been without their pressures, however, and while half of the survey respondents felt that being in the PDU did not in itself make their work more difficult, an equal number expressed the view that there was never enough time to spend on such activity. Certainly, as time has passed resources have become increasingly tight and such pressures have increased, making effective leadership and careful prioritisation and evaluation of work increasingly important.

So much of healthcare work and in particular that of medical wards necessitates effective inter-disciplinary communication, and the complexities of patient care benefit from an approach where all can collaborate and contribute freely . While at times increasing the expectations and pressures on staff, the developments within the PDU have encouraged a growth of confidence within members of the team, have encouraged greater mutual respect and have done much to overcome traditional barriers between professions. In doing so, they have helped to create an environment where effective healthcare and innovation in practice are more likely to succeed.

Multidisciplinary innovation

The basic purpose of the PDU is to provide an environment where innovation in multidisciplinary practice can take place, and where new approaches can be tested and evaluated. It was recognised that in order to achieve lasting change within the unit, there was a need not only to concentrate on specific individual projects, but also to focus on the culture within the unit which would enable such projects to be identified, initiated and supported. The culture aimed for by the unit's leaders was one where the needs of the patient and the quality of care offered within the unit were at the centre of any developments; which emphasised the multidisciplinary, multiagency nature of healthcare; where individual members of staff could become actively involved in debates and developments; and where critical review and evaluation of practice and a view of change as a positive phenomenon were the norm.

The approaches, already described, to 'empowering' the unit's staff were the essential foundations of this environment. This was supported by the unit's active networking with others and its drive towards the development of an evidence-based approach to care through its research and audit related activity. In addition to these aspects, however, the unit also concentrated its activity at a level which might be considered to be much more basic, but which is no less important.

The most fundamental issue was the creation and support of forums where non-threatening, multidisciplinary debate about important issues in practice could take place. In such forums, the aim was to facilitate critical reflection on practice and on new developments, to focus on interfaces between professions in patient care, and to provide a mechanism for identifying and initiating new, innovative approaches.

Initially, this was addressed by the creation of multidisciplinary management meetings and discussions on specific problems in clinical practice. The role of the unit's Clinical Leader was crucial here, as someone not perceived to be 'fighting for' any one profession and whose role was to facilitate open and democratic discussion. The use of generic 'off-the-shelf' audit tools such as Monitor (Goldstone et al., 1984) helped to engender a critical approach to practice at the outset. However, the unidisciplinary and generic nature of such tools was recognised at an early stage and while uniprofessional audit continued in parallel, in recognition of the unique aspects of professional activity, these were complemented by a focus on standard setting and audit within the unit as a multidisciplinary activity. Work on multidisciplinary standards focused on specific practice issues identified by the multidisciplinary team, including subjects such as: discharge planning, meal presentation, last offices, personalised and communal clothing, use of cot sides and single sex bedrooms. This work, together with the early focus on multidisciplinary communication and record keeping, was pivotal in establishing future working methods and relationships. While the subject matter of the standards and audit was itself important, the value of such work in promoting better understanding of roles, creating trust and developing a sense of teamwork in tackling specific local practice issues cannot be over-estimated.

As the unit continued to develop, this focus on project work involving more than one discipline was maintained. Projects were selected and prioritised with reference both to their potential to enhance patient care and to the extent to which they would continue to reinforce the multidisciplinary ethos of the PDU. A key part of the role of the unit's Leader was to support this process and to facilitate the continued active involvement of different disciplines, each of which had different professional priorities and perspectives, levels of skills and knowledge in development and evaluation of practice, and constraints on time and other resources.

The implementation of the unit's weekly Clinical Forum as a regular mechanism for debating multidisciplinary practice issues helped to further support and reinforce the ethos and practical work of the PDU. This forum enabled the unit to discuss and address specific problems at the interfaces between professions, to identify potential innovations in practice, to plan the team's approach to their implementation, and to review the results of existing developments. In addition, it allowed the unit to import new ideas from outside, via invited external speakers.

Naturally, each meeting tended to have different levels of representation from the various professions, as some subject matter naturally appealed more to certain professional groups than to others. As constraints on resources increased, the impact on the Clinical Forum also grew, with some of the less numerous professional groups having to prioritise their time increasingly in order to meet patients' needs. The role of the Leader was important in ensuring that this did not result in the increasing dominance of the forum by nurses and pure nursing issues. The maintenance of the Clinical Forum and other multidisciplinary activity needed constant attention and hard work over years in order to ensure their survival in the face of ever increasing day-to-day pressures. In spite of various ups and downs, this was largely achieved, with professionals from across the disciplines recognising the value of such forums and working very hard to ensure that they could participate.

One area where less success was achieved than the unit's leaders would have liked, was in the involvement of medical staff in the unit's multidisciplinary activities. A number of doctors took an active role in specific project work, and would certainly participate in multidisciplinary debates when invited, often contributing valuable ideas and information. Overall, however, the majority of senior medical staff within the unit's wards have seen the PDU's developmental work as largely the province of nurses and 'professions allied to medicine', with medical development and research as a separate issue. The PDU's leaders identified the potential of the recent growth in clinical audit to engage medical colleagues more closely in multidisciplinary debates and developments and the unit has therefore played a key role in the practical development of clinical audit within its hospital. While some success was achieved through this means, the issue of integrating medical and other multidisciplinary development remains a real one. The newly emerging focus on clinical effectiveness and evidence-based healthcare might provide a vehicle for continuing progress in this area.

The multidisciplinary forums and action-planning approach adopted by the PDU have enabled it to achieve notable success in the wide range of developmental work discussed in earlier chapters. Much of this work has been implemented more widely across the unit's own organisation, in addition to being publicised via journals, conferences and visits to the unit.

The unit's annual action plan has helped to focus this project work, so that the limited resources of the unit were not dissipated across too wide a field of activity. Initially, this action plan was developed as an almost entirely 'bottom-up' exercise, with facilitation by the Leader and managers of the unit. As time progressed, in order to enable the unit to build on the foundations of its earlier work, to increase the rigour of PDU projects, and to focus ever-tighter resources more sharply, the open, 'bottom-up' agenda setting was balanced with the identification of a small number of clear priorities for the unit – such as continued development of multidisciplinary records, stroke care, and Dealing Decently with Death. For the year 1996/7, there were nevertheless still 28 clinical objectives, causing some questions to be asked about the feasibility of such a programme. To some extent such questions were justified in the light of the forthcoming hospital merger and its accompanying radical management restructuring, the profound effects of which on the development of practice could not be foreseen when the plan was set. However, there is also a need to understand the different rationales behind the publication of such a programme within the unit. While being primarily an explicit plan of action, it also functions as a demonstration of the breadth of current work for those outside the unit, and within the unit as a means of celebrating current work and of rewarding individuals identified as project leaders. In addition, it serves as a practical tool to reinforce the identity and multidisciplinary ethos of the unit and to demonstrate that individuals can indeed influence its agenda. Therefore, while not all projects may be concluded successfully, the value of the plan also needs to be measured in other ways. There has always been a tension in the unit's action planning between the maintenance of a realistic programme and the promotion and positive demonstration of a high level of staff involvement.

A proportion of failures along the way has always been accepted in the unit, where the aims are to try out new ideas and to encourage people to involve themselves in managed risk taking. The challenge for the unit's leaders has been to balance this with the need to achieve real, well planned developments and to build the rigour and complexity of the unit's work over time on the foundation of earlier work.

Research

From its inception, the PDU has espoused the idea of evidence-based healthcare. The unit has promoted an approach to care which reflects the true multidisciplinary nature of such care, and which is based on the use of the best available knowledge. Within its bounds, the unit has fostered a critical approach which has valued and supported reflection, continuous audit of practice and the application of research and other evidence into the practice setting. In more recent years, the unit also aimed to carry out selected practice-based research which reflected its multidisciplinary ethos and expertise.

Narrowing the theory–practice gap was an important early priority of the unit, and this was always an important priority within the role of the PDU Leader. Development of skills and knowledge in appreciation and evaluation of research was seen as an essential underpinning to innovation in practice. The clinical debates taking place within the unit offered staff the opportunity to critically examine their practice and to consider it in the light of research-based evidence. In addition, access to formal education programmes, both in-house and external, was combined with other more flexible, practice-based approaches, such as structured involvement in the various aspects of the unit's project work. Such practice-based learning opportunities helped to ensure that the use of research in practice was embedded in the normal routines of the unit, rather than being perceived as something related primarily to formal education. The support provided for staff through the Research Advisory Group (RAG) also helped to raise the profile of research within the unit, and offered staff a high level of expert advice and information both to help them effectively evaluate specific developmental work and to develop skills in appreciation and appraisal of research evidence.

The importance of basing clinical practice guidelines on research evidence had been realised at Seacroft before the PDU was created. The Nursing Clinical Practice Group, to which the first PDU Clinical Leader contributed, had been particularly active in producing guidance for nurses on a range of topics. Other professions were also actively using research to influence the development of their practice. What the PDU managed to do was to bring everyone together in ways which enabled each profession to share specialist knowledge in critically evaluating practice and in developing evidence-based approaches to care which were multidisciplinary in focus.

Later, the development of clinical audit as a means of addressing the multidisciplinary nature of healthcare and of supporting a research culture, was eagerly embraced by the PDU. Seacroft Hospital was fortunate in having professionals who were willing to expose their audit work to open scrutiny and debate. The multidisciplinary approach of the PDU and its routine use of audit in practice were fundamental in building on this foundation across the whole hospital. In the early stages of clinical audit development, the Leader of the PDU collaborated with the Practice Development Nurse of an associated hospital in obtaining a regional grant to develop a framework for nursing and therapy audit across the organisation. Initially, this resulted in conflict between the new development of the nursing and therapy audit and the established medical audit infrastructure. From this initial conflict, however, arose a hospital-wide, collaborative approach to clinical audit involving all disciplines. Such a transformation was almost momentous in scale, representing a major shift in attitude and behaviour within the hospital, and it was the ethos and the drive of the PDU which was largely responsible for bringing this about.

Within this new approach, regular clinical audit forums provided a vehicle for analysing and debating multidisciplinary practice issues involving all disciplines, including medicine. This approach further reinforced the emphasis on evidence and its use in practice within the unit, and also provided a mechanism through which the PDU could influence other areas of the hospital.

Recently, there has been a growth of interest in evidence-based practice, meaning that treatment and care should as far as possible be based upon research evidence of effectiveness (Long and Harrison, 1996). Contrary to what is probably the prevailing lay view, knowledge of what works best in healthcare is still developing and there is much work yet to do in ensuring that such knowledge is put into practice.

The PDU had been addressing these sorts of issues some time before phrases like clinical effectiveness achieved their current profile on the NHS agenda. The basic thrust of the PDU approach is that it is usually only possible to deliver effective heathcare if all involved in the team work well together. The PDU sees effectiveness as a much wider concept than just one of saying 'which treatment works best?'. It is also important to consider how such treatments are applied in the complex healthcare environment. The most important contributions of the PDU to the application of research lie in the unit's ability to create a climate where reflection on practice and the critical review of practice in the light of research and other evidence are the norm, and where sophisticated approaches to the implementation of research evidence can be developed which reflect the real complexity and multiagency nature of healthcare practice.

Once the PDU was well established, it aimed also to develop a programme of clinically-focused research within its own confines. The difficulty of establishing rigorous research activity cannot be stressed enough. Research needs resources in terms of people and time. It is expecting a lot of heavily committed clinical staff to find the time for research too. With this in mind, the PDU developed from an existing role the post of Research Practitioner. In addition to providing essential support for the continued development of the use of research in practice, the Research Practitioner was seen as the key to the development of a formal research profile. The PDU had already proven itself very successful in finding and creating opportunities for evaluating practice with very limited resources. However, the development of a programme of formal research projects was a further step for the unit.

Reflecting its own strengths and the principles of the emerging NHS R&D strategy, the PDU aimed to focus on very specific projects where it had already undertaken successful developmental work. In addition, it aimed to develop partnerships, primarily through the Research Practitioner, with other healthcare providers and with academics, in order to increase the quality of such work and the likelihood of acceptance of any funding proposals.

With this in mind the unit pursued two specific projects – the investigation into the education and information needs of newly diagnosed diabetic patients, and research into physiotherapy in stroke patients. The former involved a collaboration between the PDU and a local university, and was resourced by both the university itself and by PDU trust funds which enabled the release of a research nurse. The second was the subject of a successful grant application by the Research Practitioner to the regional NHS Executive office. This was the only work within the unit which was funded by formal research moneys, as opposed to audit and practice development grants or other 'soft' funding.

The unit had successfully completed the first stage in its progress onto the research ladder and the hope was that such successful small projects would increase the chances when bidding for larger grants later. Successful bidders needed a reputation for managing grants well. The PDU had succeeded in gaining much needed experience in applying for grants, putting proposals to research ethics committees and running projects. Unfortunately, because of the broader circumstances of the unit, it was not possible to develop this initial research work further.

In terms of carrying out research, as opposed to using it in practice or using some of its methods in evaluation of developmental work, the PDU can claim only limited success. A few people were involved in research from time to time. Most were not involved, and it was never intended that this should be the case. What did evolve was a growing acceptance that research was relevant and important. A culture was successfully created within the PDU where questioning rather than acceptance was the norm, where reflection on practice and considered application of evidence to practice were everyday events. In addition to this, the PDU successfully developed the skills and knowledge base of a large cross-section of its workforce, rather than just a selected few individuals, which enabled this type of activity to take place. This emphasis on the use of research within the PDU and the unit's success in the different aspects of research work were reflected in a survey of staff views (Allsopp and Page, 1995). While a relatively disappointing number of staff felt that carrying out research within the unit was of fairly low priority, over half mentioned research in their definition of what a PDU was, and most expressed the view that the dissemination and use of research were a high priority.

The final issue to consider in a review of research within the PDU is in its use to evaluate the unit itself. From the outset the need to demonstrate the value of the unit and its work through careful evaluation was explicitly identified as one of the aims of the unit. In addition to its clinical importance, such evaluation is essential as a means of satisfying managers that scarce resources are being used wisely, as well as demonstrating to the staff themselves what they have achieved. The PDU approach was to insist that all new projects be properly planned and have clear aims and objectives. It took a while to learn this lesson, however. People with an idea just want to get on with it and change everything. They can take some persuading to stop and clarify what it is they are wanting to change in specific terms and then to agree a method and process for evaluating the change. Delays can then mean a loss of momentum, and sometimes a loss of enthusiasm.

Nevertheless, a significant amount of data has been collected over the years, which can be used to evaluate the performance of the unit. On a basic level, this relates to the degree to which it has achieved the objectives stated in its action plan. Beyond this, evaluation data have been gathered related to the implementation and effectiveness of most of the individual projects initiated within the unit, which can offer a clear picture of many of the unit's achievements.

However, where the unit has achieved less success has been in the use of formal research to evaluate differences between its own culture and quality of care and those in other clinical areas. Anecdotal evidence within the hospital clearly identified the unit as different and superior to other clinical settings in its multidisciplinary and patient-centred approach. The sheer level of developmental activity taking place and level of influence exerted by this across the organisation were also visibly different to other areas, and out of all proportion to the unit's geographical size or physical resources. The survey of staff views carried out in 1995 (Allsopp and Page, 1995) demonstrated that in spite of the growing resource pressures and the difficulty of maintaining the PDU's activity, the majority of its staff at all grades felt that the unit was different to other areas they had worked in and provided an environment which was conducive to their personal development and involvement, and to innovation in patient care. That these views should prevail not just in a few key staff, but across the majority of the team, can be held to be a key achievement of the unit.

However, an attempt to evaluate the culture in comparison to other wards within the hospital's Department of Medicine using the Team Climate Inventory (Anderson and West, 1994) produced less conclusive results. While it was felt that this tool would provide a useful means of evaluating the desired culture within the PDU, being based in part on some of the literature which had influenced the unit's own development, a number of other difficulties affected the study. Primarily these included the difficulty for many practitioners in interpreting questions which referred to their 'team'. While most staff within the PDU perceived themselves to be a part of the PDU team, all also legitimately considered themselves at other times to be a part of at least one other team – for example, primary nurse team, physiotherapy team, ward team. A further possible influence related to the fact that the comparison wards were adjacent to the PDU and part of the same department. Over the years, while not explicitly part of the unit, much collaboration had taken place between the two areas and many of the opportunities created by the PDU were also shared with staff on the other wards. This was particularly the case in recent years, where the unit's aims explicitly included the influencing of other areas. Indeed, in 1996 the unit was formally expanded to include the other wards in the Department of Medicine. Because of these issues, while the results of the study were useful in discussion with the respective staff groups, they were not felt to have helped in the overall evaluation of the unit.

The most ambitious research-related project attempted by the unit reflected this need to provide hard, comparative evidence of the value of the PDU approach. What was required was felt to be a formal research study, led by an expert team of external researchers, which would compare key outcomes of the PDU with those of other non-PDU areas of a similar size and with comparable clinical caseloads and resources. The possibility of such a study was explored with a team from the University of York. The response of the York team to the unit's approach was very encouraging, and several meetings took place aimed at agreeing some form of research strategy and trying to find funding. The idea of a randomised trial was discussed, in which patient outcomes would be compared between those admitted to PDU wards and others admitted to non-PDU wards at Seacroft. However, other similar units were needed to take part and in spite of considerable effort over a number of months, none could be found that were both comparable to the PDU and able to randomise patient admissions in this way. To complicate matters further, one of the PDU's ward managers moved to a non-PDU comparison ward within the hospital's Department of Medicine and discussions were taking place about amalgamating the planned control wards into the PDU, and these factors further exacerbated the researchers' problem of 'contamination' of control wards already discussed in relation to the Team Climate Inventory. For these reasons, it was therefore inevitable that the plans had to be abandoned. This experience highlights very clearly the extreme difficulty of conducting this sort of research. The PDU had been very successful at demonstrating the benefits of individual projects, but whether patients 'did better' by being admitted to a PDU must unfortunately remain unknown because of the the multiple problems of conducting a detailed and rigorous study in such a complex and continuously changing environment.

Patient empowerment

One of the central tenets of the PDU approach is its focus on the users of the service – patients, carers and others. This central focus has overwhelmingly driven the activity of the PDU. It has ensured a focus on the processes of care as a whole, rather than on the function of individual departments or professional groups. In doing so, it has cut across traditional boundaries and has managed to exert an influence in ways which the more common uniprofessional or departmentally led approaches to development are unable to realise. The unit's approach is consistent with many of the principles of quality management theory, and any managers reading this book will have readily recognised this fact. Important differences between the usual approach to implementation of quality management principles and the work of the PDU, however, lie primarily in the focus on the patient as an individual which complements the abstract consideration of processes, and secondly in the human element in the application of such theory within the multidisciplinary team. By the latter, we mean the fact that while quality management and other theory may well form a part of what the PDU is about, a key part of the unit's success in implementing these things has been due to its ability to put into practice the essential elements, without recourse to the accompanying jargon which is usually alien and often offensive to healthcare professionals. Commonly, 'quality' and 'customer-focused' approaches are implemented in organisations as something entirely new and requiring a new language and supporting structures which are created in addition to any already in existence. The PDU has offered an insight into how such approaches can be implemented into a real health service setting, without alienating professional teams and without the creation of a new department.

Much of the project work within the unit has been either directly or indirectly aimed at empowering its patients and carers. The multidisciplinary records were developed explicitly with the intention of making them available and comprehensible to patients. Evaluative work was carried out on the use of these records which highlighted professional jargon which patients did not understand, and action was taken to eliminate the use of such terms. A heavy emphasis was placed upon patient education within many of the unit's projects, such as the development of self-medication, implementation of constipation protocols, and provision of discharge information in lay terms.

The evaluation of the PDU's activities and basic quality of care was routinely informed by patients' and carers' views. From the outset, this was based around the use of questionnaires to obtain views on aspects of the service and to measure 'satisfaction'. As time progressed, the unit grew aware of the need to develop more sophisticated approaches to eliciting users' views in order to supplement such statistical data, and techniques of individual interviewing and use of focus groups were introduced. The recent project employing the focus group technique to investigate diabetic patients' and carers' perceptions of their need for information, education and support after their initial diagnosis was particularly successful. This opened up new possibilities for the unit to complement the research and theoretical evidence and practical expertise of its practitioners which underpinned its work, with the detailed experiences of individual patients – an important milestone on the road to real 'evidence-based' healthcare.

The PDU was established with a fundamental belief in the importance of informing, involving and empowering its patients. From a relatively simple start, the unit consistently maintained its belief in this principle, which informed virtually all of its practical work in one way or another. The sophistication of the unit's approaches also continued to develop over time, with new possibilities opening up with the discovery and espousal of more recently introduced techniques. The majority of those treated on the PDU probably had no idea that they were on a PDU as opposed to any other type of ward. However, the many investigations into views of patients conducted over the years, together with the feedback from other professionals in a position to form a judgement (such as the discharge liaison nurses), have left no doubt that while the unit was always aware that more work could be done, it consistently provided a very positive and actively supportive environment for its patients.

Networking

When it was first established, firm links were forged between the PDU and a local university. The value of such a collaboration was seen in the PDU as something which would be of benefit both to the unit itself and to its academic partners. The unit placed great emphasis on the development of its staff, and the inclusion of professional educators within the PDU team helped to ensure that educational developments implemented within the unit were innovative and based on sound theory. The PDU also needed to be able to evaluate its work with a degree of rigour if it was to be taken seriously. The contributions of academic partners in this regard were extremely important to the unit, particularly in its early stages when such skills were still relatively scarce within the unit itself.

The PDU linked particularly well with nursing lecturers at Leeds Metropolitan University (LMU), and with the College of Health in

Leeds, later to merge with the School of Healthcare Studies at Leeds University. These lecturers were very supportive in their work for the PDU RAG, and also played a significant role in later collaborations related to specific project work. PDU and other Seacroft staff also contributed to various courses at LMU from time to time, linking with academic staff from a range of other university departments.

The PDU was fortunate, particularly in its early years, to have a regional health authority which included some very enlightened people supporting practice development. PDU links with the nursing directorate at 'Region' were to develop when the Institute of Nursing at Leeds University was created. The nursing directorate had accredited the PDU in 1993 and this link was to be fruitful later as PDU staff were able to provide an input into the work of the Institute through its practice development network forums and research and development network. PDU staff were also invited to write and teach a module on the Institute's Master's programme on Therapeutic Nursing.

The benefits, of course, were not just for the PDU. University departments need clinical areas in which to place students of all types. It is to the advantage of students also to work in the sort of culture the PDU provides. Many student nurses deliberately chose to return to work at Seacroft because of their PDU experience. In addition, universities need access to clinical areas for research and in order to ground their theoretical teaching. Having a PDU in which the climate is very supportive towards research and towards innovation in multidisciplinary practice can only be to the advantage of university staff.

As well as linking with higher education, the value of partnerships with other organisations was also realised. Perhaps the most important of these are the community health and social services on which so many of the patients going through the PDU come to depend on discharge from hospital. Discharge planning formed a key part of PDU project work which helped Seacroft to maintain its fine reputation for effective discharge planning. Liaison between the medical service and community services was good, and the feedback received in the PDU from district nursing staff was largely very positive. The appointment of a community liaison nurse based part time in the PDU itself has already demonstrated benefits in improved working arrangements and collaboration between primary and secondary care. A whole month of PDU Clinical Forum meetings devoted to discussions of primary/secondary care 'interface' issues showed just what could be done.

Other links were established between the PDU and Leeds Carers' Centre. Again, the siting of the leader of this project at Seacroft, with a resource area in the PDU, helped raise the profile of carers' issues and facilitated collaboration with the existing Carers' Support Group led by the PDU's own staff.

Working with another Trust in Liverpool on a clinical supervision project gave the unit an opportunity to explore new avenues for development. One of the aims of the collaboration was to see if such a networking arrangement could actually be valuable to both trusts in moving forward on a particular issue. Although this project was unfortunately not seen through to a successful conclusion, both because of difficulties associated with the complexity of the subject matter and the practical problems of the networking itself, significant lessons were learned and benefits gained by both partners in the collaboration.

In Chapter 10 both the positive and negative sides of networking were discussed. If care is not taken in its implementation, the activity can strengthen a view of a unit as elitist and foster feelings of alienation among staff left out of the process. In addition, it can be expensive in both time and money and if not managed carefully and integrated into the broader aims and approaches of the unit can rightly be perceived as wasteful and luxurious. The PDU was generally successful in avoiding these pitfalls and integrated its use of networking carefully into its other developmental work, so that it both benefited a wide range of individuals as part of the unit's approach to staff empowerment, and contributed positively to specific practice development work and its dissemination.

Dissemination

The unit placed a heavy emphasis on the need to share its work with others. This it has done very successfully over the years, both through formal channels and through informal networking arrangements.

The unit began its dissemination endeavours on a relatively small scale internally through publication of reports and provision of education sessions, and externally through seminars and conference presentations at events facilitated by the regional nursing department. From these presentations, staff from other organisations began to request visits to the PDU in order to discuss both the theoretical underpinning of the unit and its support, and to see how it worked in practice. Over the subsequent years, the unit has received hundreds of visitors and posted out a vast number of reports and copies of its newly developed documentation.

In recent years, the sophistication of the unit's approach to dissemination has developed considerably. More recently, it distinguished between the approaches used for external dissemination, where the aim was principally to share information and ideas to stimulate debates on practice, and those adopted for dissemination within its own organisation, where in addition to sharing of ideas the aim was increasingly to directly influence specific practices and/or the overall culture in another clinical area.

In the area of external dissemination, the unit developed more efficient and targeted approaches to information sharing, and also sought to publish its work in as wide a range of journals and conferences as possible, to reflect the breadth of those who might be interested in the PDU approach – nurses, managers, therapists, doctors and others. Its own conference and exhibition events also proved successful in attracting a multidisciplinary audience and in opening up debate across the disciplines.

With regard to internal dissemination, the unit developed new working partnerships with other clinical teams within the organisation. Rather than completing project work solely within the confines of the PDU and then attempting to 'sell' it to other practitioners as a finished product, developmental projects were planned collaboratively between the PDU and others, in order to ensure their relevance to other clinical settings and to promote their ownership and uptake by those outside the unit. This was a far cry from the standard development unit approach which not uncommonly resulted in accusations of elitism from those outside and the development of an automatic resistance to their ideas. Broader success from such collaborations included the further development of the unit's multidisciplinary records and the Dealing Decently with Death project, both of which influenced the whole hospital. Unfortunately, it was not possible to measure the extent to which such collaborations successfully influenced the culture and working patterns of other areas.

A considerable regret of the PDU's leaders is the extent to which they failed to take up opportunities for evaluation of their external dissemination. With the exception of statistical data on numbers of visits, reports distributed and papers published and presented, the unit has no clear idea of the impact of its work on the wider world. It has received many messages of thanks from those visiting and making inquiries, expressing the degree to which the information and insight provided by the team have been found helpful. In addition, a number of units have progressed after visiting the PDU to seek development unit accreditation themselves. However, no clear data have ever been collected to determine the precise uses to which information provided by the PDU has been put. Have similar practice developments been introduced elsewhere based on PDU work? Did the unit's work influence the philosophy or culture established elsewhere? Has it stimulated the development of a more multidisciplinary approach to practice in other hospitals? Unfortunately we will never know. A clear message then for others embarking on a similar venture is to aim from the outset to follow up inquiries, visits or presentations, and to seek information on uptake of ideas and new practices.

Overall, in spite of this regret about the extent to which its dissemination was formally evaluated, the PDU has been effective in disseminating its work. Without a doubt its reputation as a centre for innovation was out of proportion to its actual size and the resources at its disposal, and this was based not on flashy presentational techniques, but on real work carried out within the unit. The work of the unit in this regard gives a clear indication of what can be achieved with even limited resources when the climate and support within the organisation are right.

The PDU in context

The PDU was established at least in part to facilitate the integration of two hospital teams. The aim was to create one effective new department, where staff from the two very different settings would work closely together as one team, and towards the same goals. It was recognised that elements of good practice existed on both sites which ought to be maintained and carried forward. However, it was also important to ensure that the new unit would not be encumbered with historical baggage, but would be seen as something quite distinct from what had gone before. While continuing to celebrate the positive elements of the existing structure, the desire was to create a climate within the new team where change and the introduction and testing of new ideas would be perceived as the norm, and viewed as positive phenomena. The newly emerging NDU approach was recognised as a potential vehicle for such a change, but the experience of the effective multidisciplinary culture at St George's Hospital combined with an awareness of recently published quality and other management theory created a dissatisfaction with an approach which concentrated on one discipline only, and this resulted in the conception of the PDU as a distinct approach. Therefore, while indirectly influenced by theory from a variety of sources which was synthesised by its original leaders, the PDU also largely arose from a specific set of circumstances and resulted in the creation and refinement of a model of practice and its development which was carefully tailored to suit these circumstances.

From the successful pragmatism of this early development, the unit's leaders were able to proceed to a clearer definition of the PDU 'model', including its philosophy and key features, aims and objectives, mode of working and systems of support. This model proved itself extremely valuable in continuing to galvanise the unit's team and to focus it on positive development after the loss of the initial impetus arising from the hospital merger. This initial momentum was maintained and increased with the greater definition of the model and the extent to which the unit's staff identified with and 'owned' it. At this early stage, while it brought with it its own problems, the accreditation process offered by the Yorkshire Region was invaluable: as a vehicle within the unit for critically evaluating progress towards its goals, as a means of strengthening the external focus on the unit and of lending it an additional credibility both within the unit and in the larger organisation arising from its external endorsement. The associated opportunities for networking were also vital to the unit both in exposing its own team to a breadth of new ideas, and also in building the confidence and enthusiasm of the staff through opportunities to celebrate and share their own good work and to discuss issues with others of like mind. This period resulted in notable successes for the unit in specific project work, consolidation of the PDU model in practice, and in a recognition of the broader applicability of the PDU approach to other healthcare settings. The PDU became a source of information to many around the region and beyond who wished to create similar climates for multidisciplinary innovation within their own organisations.

After this early period of relative stability, the unit's circumstances continued to change and a further merger took place between the PDU's own and another hospital. This was a time of great instability in the broader environment, which was further exacerbated by a significant change in the key personnel within the unit. In addition, the priorities of the health service as a whole continued to shift, with an increasing emphasis on value for money and on rigorous clinical evaluation, through the development of the NHS R&D strategy and introduction of Clinical Audit. During this period the unit's leaders recognised that the survival of the PDU depended on its ability to maintain its essential identity, as defined by its philosophy and essential elements, but to adapt its approach to work and systems of support to meet the new challenges. It was also essential to demonstrate clearly both the rigour of the the unit's work and its value in concrete terms to the broader organisation. During this period, the role of PDU Leader evolved away from its initial primarily clinical focus and towards a greater emphasis on change management and facilitation skills. The political skills of the Leader were also of increasing importance at this time, as the environment within which the unit operated became more politically charged and management structures more fluid. The role of Research Practitioner was introduced in order to support the development of increased rigour in evaluation of the unit's work and to begin to increase the level of research activity within the unit. The uncertainty created by the unit's external circumstances resulted in severe difficulty at times in maintaining the motivation of the unit's team. However, the strength and adaptability of the PDU model and the degree to which it was believed in by the staff, enabled the unit to emerge from this difficult period not only with a programme of project work firmly integrated into the business plans of the organisation as a whole, but also with a much clearer understanding of the PDU model, its value to an organisation, and its potential for adaptation and use in a variety of circumstances.

More recently, the PDU's hospital has undergone a further merger, this time with a much larger teaching hospital trust. The management structure of the hospital underwent further considerable change and it was necessary to adapt the PDU Leader role to function in a new, less directly supported environment where the unit's managers were at a greater distance from the unit itself and directly responsible for a significantly larger patch. During this time, the unit continued its programme of developments and also involved itself in trust-wide debates and developments, successfully bringing to bear its philosophy for multidisciplinary empowerment and innovation on the more traditionally oriented agenda of the larger organisation – both in the arena of clinical practice development and audit and that of broader organisational quality issues. The unit also sought to broaden its boundaries to include the other wards within Seacroft Hospital. The rationale for this lay in the belief that the value of the unit lay not only in its ability to influence specific aspects of practice in other areas, but also to influence the overall culture.

Within the unit itself, successful practice development continued. However, there was difficulty in maintaining the developmental momentum because of the level of organisational uncertainty and lack of tangible support from the department's managers, whose attention was necessarily elsewhere. In the event, this difficulty was compounded by the larger scale of the unit, which tended to dilute the level of support which could be provided by the unit's leaders.

In more stable circumstances, the physical expansion of the PDU might have proven successful. However, at the conclusion of the merger process, the PDU ultimately became part of an even larger Division of Medicine, which formed approximately one third of the whole trust. It was felt important within the new organisation to create a division-wide approach to practice development, which focused on development and implementation of specific policies and procedures. It was apparent that the PDU model as it existed was not suited to directly sustaining practice development on this scale or with this specific focus.

The approach which is emerging within the division is one which seeks to marry together the Trust's existing centralised but unidisciplinary models of practice development, research and audit with the more integrative and multidisciplinary approach demanded by the recent clinical effectiveness movement. While the inability of the PDU to survive the merger in its original form has been a source of considerable disappointment to its staff, its ideas and the experience of its team have exerted a significant influence on the new approach adopted within the division (of 500 beds on three sites) and on its application in practice. This can be argued to be no small achievement for a unit based around three hospital wards.

The PDU and the accreditation process

The PDU was heavily influenced by criteria for NDUs set out by both the King's Fund and the Nursing Directorate at Yorkshire Region, later to become the Centre for the Development of Nursing Policy and Practice at Leeds University ('The Centre').

As previously discussed, the PDUs accreditation by Yorkshire Region was valuable in that it provided the PDU with an external, independent view of what was happening at Seacroft, with specific goals to work towards, with access to valuable networks and with an external endorsement which was equally useful in raising the belief in the unit both within its own confines and among the organisation's managers. Not only was the PDU the first unit to gain success in accreditation, but it was also the first multidisciplinary unit to be recognised by what was principally a nursing development unit scheme. This said something about the strength of the model (as well as the powers of persuasion of PDU leaders). It also set the scene for what was to be an ongoing debate between the PDU and the accreditation team as to the meaning of a scheme which focused on just one profession, i.e. nursing.

The very nature of the PDU and its multidisciplinary focus made accreditation a difficult process. As the PDU itself developed it became increasingly clear that the criteria no longer seemed to fit. The PDU was growing in sophistication and adapting to new circumstances within its organisation, while the accreditation criteria appeared rigid and inflexible. Discussions with 'The Centre' continued for three years or more, as change engulfed both the trust and the university. The PDU was never reaccredited, and this was not seen as a problem within the unit, as the model developed within the PDU itself was felt to have become sufficiently robust and distinct from that of the accreditation scheme for such reaccreditation to be superfluous. In particular, the multidisciplinary nature of the PDU and its integration into the organisation's wider business plans sat very uncomfortably with the nursing focus of the accreditation scheme and its demand for a separate 'business plan'.

It was understandably difficult for what was an organisation aimed at developing nursing and nurses to openly declare a multidisciplinary philosophy. The PDU and 'The Centre' had very good relations, but it is only fair to say that at times there was a certain distance in thinking between the two. One of the issues was what the PDU was getting for any possible future payment for reaccreditation or evaluation. The experience of the first year after initial accreditation had been one of very little support from 'The Centre' (or the Institute, as it was then). This was partly due to changes in key personnel, but also appeared to represent a lack of appreciation of what was expected. For the PDU, finding the money to pay for reaccreditation was a big issue. Managers were wanting value for money and this had to be made clear. At the least there should be some form of ongoing support for development units once accreditation had been achieved. This might include staff and team development support, and help with evaluation of work for instance. The dialogue between the PDU and 'The Centre' was in the end a constructive one, and the PDU was able to influence the refashioning of the accreditation process. This process and the contribution of the PDU to its development are discussed below.

- **Stage 1** is achieved when the nursing or practice development unit successfully fulfils the criteria (see Chapter 3) and their potential for development is apparent.
- **Stage 2** is awarded to those teams who have not only fulfilled the scheme's criteria, but who can demonstrate they are disseminating evaluated practice to nurses and the professions allied to medicine. In addition those teams who have opted to become practice development units need to demonstrate that collaboration between professional groups is truly enacted and not just something to which lip service is paid.

What happens after accreditation is less well defined. Having achieved stage 2, NDU and PDU staff are required to submit annual reports detailing their progress. In the past this has assured their accreditation status. As more and more units join the scheme it has become increasingly apparent that the accreditation team needed to design a systematic and robust follow-up. It was considered this would add rigour to the process, but more importantly, would maintain the high profile of the NDU or PDU in the organisation.

The form that follow-up should take was a matter for discussion between 'The Centre' and members of the practice development network around the region, and in particular the representatives of the PDU. It was agreed that a form of evaluation was preferable to reaccreditation. The notion of reaccreditation against set criteria was felt to be too rigid to apply to units which were designed to push at the boundaries of current practice, and which needed to be able to adapt freely to changing organisational circumstances. Once the basic level of achievement represented by accreditation had been achieved, it was felt that such an approach would tend to restrict rather than encourage innovation within the development units. It was important to have an evaluation framework that was meaningful and relevant to contemporary practice. Evaluation would need to capture those issues deemed to be at the forefront of patient care, and yet would be dynamic and sensitive to changes currently affecting healthcare delivery on the ground.

Evaluation would address issues at a macro and micro level. Both approaches were considered to be of equal importance. At a macro level there was a need to evaluate the impact of the nursing and practice development unit scheme on healthcare delivery and on the leader's career paths. Some development units now have their third or fourth generation of leaders and a focus on the evaluation of career paths is an important issue in considerations of future leadership requirements and of ensuring continuity in the work of such units. On a micro level, a need was identified for evaluation to be informed by the perspectives of their various local stakeholders, asking specifically:

- what has changed?
- what has caused the change?
- how is the change affecting practice?

To support this evaluation process the development of an evaluation team was agreed, which would work with already accredited units to facilitate a biennial peer review process. This process would not only benefit the scheme, but more importantly would enhance the unit leaders' individual and professional development, thus contributing to the wider development of practice. The accreditation team and newly created evaluation team would work in parallel, but with shared aims and objectives.

Credibility of the team involved in evaluating progress within specific units is a key issue, and the composition of the team was revised to include the leaders of nursing and practice development units in the region which are accredited to stage 2 of the scheme. 'The Centre' considered that the leaders' practical experience of systematically evaluating their own progress, and in continuing to explore the basic development unit model in a variety of settings, would bring a broader perspective to the debates and would contribute to the development of future plans. The recent debates have also seen the inclusion of multidisciplinary representation in the teams, reflecting the PDU debate and the growth of interest in this approach.

'The Centre' acknowledged that the issue of sustained organisational support was an area of difficulty for units, especially post accreditation. Development units struggle if their managerial support wanes and having external commitment and external support can be invaluable in helping them to survive in what is sometimes a hostile climate. The evaluation process was considered to be an effective means of continuing to offer this level of external support and endorsement, without restricting the development of the individual units by the application of rigid criteria.

The interest in accreditation as PDU or NDU is still growing, and 'The Centre' is continuing actively to develop its scheme. For a number of years the PDU went its own way, but ultimately the dialogue between the two organisations has been a fruitful one, which has enriched both and has served to strengthen the development unit model and to broaden the appeal and applicability of the approach.

Conclusion and future prospects

What can be learned from the Seacroft experience? The PDU has been an experiment in changing NHS culture which has demonstrated real benefits in the way professionals can work closely together in achieving quality care for patients. It has initiated a broad range of specific developments in multidisciplinary clinical practice and management, the benefits of which have been realised by both the PDU's own patients and those of other departments and organisations. Beyond this, the unit has made a lasting impression on those who worked within it, and will remain a significant influence on their philosophy and practice. The unit has influenced the beliefs and approach to developmental work across its own organisation over a number of years and has hopefully also achieved a similar, if less direct effect, in other organisations and individuals which came into contact with it. Its ideas and approaches have also influenced the reshaping of a national accreditation scheme. Perhaps the published work of the unit and the ideas carried forth by the many staff who worked within it will continue to exert an influence in various settings in the future. The extent of these achievements should not be underestimated and demonstrate what can be achieved by even a small unit, with minimal funds, where the climate supports the development and motivation of the organisation's key resource – its own staff.

The PDU approach has shown itself to be adaptable to a wide variety of different organisational circumstances, and to addressing a range of issues. However, this particular unit has not been able to survive the final merger of its hospital with the local teaching hospital trust. A critical success factor for the PDU has been senior management support. Initially, the unit's managers were also its most ardent supporters. Over time, as the organisational structure flattened, the senior managers of the PDU became further removed from the everyday work of the unit itself. This increased the political significance of the Leader role and raised the importance of integrating the unit's developmental plans with the broader organisational business plan. Nevertheless, the senior managers were familiar with the PDU approach and supportive of its continuation. Following the more recent reorganisation, the unit's senior management are even further removed from the unit itself, and are immersed in the large scale concerns of the teaching hospital. In addition, therapy services reverted to a central management structure, which to some extent cut across the integrated approach developed within the unit. Debates took place within the new division as to the best way to take forward practice development. The continued support of the PDU and its integration into a broader divisional approach was one possible way forward. However, in the event, while the ideas of the PDU were influential, this model was rejected in favour of one more familiar to those operating within the teaching hospital setting, and perceived to be more likely to be cost effective in supporting specific change across the division over the short term.

It may be that development units represent a 'phase' in the development of health service organisational culture. The real achievement is in having tried, and succeeded for a time, to show how things could be better. The rapidly changing demands of healthcare require service providers which can be flexible and adaptable in their response, and can even map out new routes as yet untested. The size, structure and culture of large hospital trusts seems to militate against such responsiveness. The analogy of a large oil tanker taking five miles to stop and change direction has been drawn. If large hospitals are to adapt as organisations there is a need for all of them to address the issue of organisational culture. If they are to get the most out of their staff, if they want a workforce which can think for itself in tackling problems sensibly and creatively, if they want to provide the best for patients, then they must work on providing the sort of culture which transforms people and constantly renews motivation. Such changes in culture, flexibility and innovation in practice can much more readily be achieved in small units. However, this virtue of small units and their potential benefits over the longer term has somehow to be balanced with the desire for economies of scale and the need to exert rapid influence on specific practice issues across whole organisations. Some form of federal structure which provides central direction, purpose and sets corporate standards, coupled with flexible local units, may be the answer.

One of the great ironies of the loss of the PDU at this point; is the rise at the same time of the debate about clinical effectiveness and evidence-based practice. Recent NHS white papers (DOH, 1996a,b) have actively sought to promote an emphasis on multidisciplinary, evidence-based care, and the more active involvement of service users in decision-making processes. Furthermore, there is a growing view that the achievement of clinical effectiveness is not simply a matter of applying clear-cut research evidence into a neutral and readily accessible practice environment. Rather, while changing knowledge may be a relatively straightforward exercise, the implementation of new knowledge into practice involves a consideration also of the specific context of practice. This includes the physical circumstances, resources available, the political agendas within the organisation, and most importantly, given the multiagency nature of healthcare, the attitudes and behaviour of staff from all disciplines within the team. As one recent paper puts it:

> Clinicians are the real agents of change. Engaging all the appropriate players in the initial process is essential. Increasingly, clinical guidelines have a multiprofessional emphasis and impact, and require appropriate interprofessional involvement. (Humphris and Littlejohns, 1996)

The common ground between the debate on achieving clinical effectiveness and the PDU approach does not end with the concept of multidisciplinary working, however. Another recent paper identifies that 'whatever its use, the uptake of evidence requires professional staff with up-to-date knowledge and skills as well as appropriate attitudes. They need to work together in cohesive and collaborative clinical teams which support them to meet both patients' and strategic needs.' (Batstone and Edwards, 1996b). The paper proceeds to consider the importance of integrating developmental and clinical audit work, and of linking the two closely into the business cycle. It concludes that:

> Perhaps a long term goal of participation in a project approach to evidence based practice lies in the potential for a cultural change in an organisation. . . .

The clinical effectiveness debate is now mirroring closely many of the concerns of the PDU over recent years. The recent emphasis on clinical effectiveness has also brought with it a fresh debate about the integration of healthcare work not only across departments and disciplines, but also across organisations. New approaches to planning and 'contracting for' health services are being debated which reflect this change of emphasis from the relatively narrow view of isolated episodes of care carried out within individual organisations, to one which considers 'streams of care' which span a variety of organisations and settings. Within a large organisation, the PDU has the potential to provide an effective vehicle for collaborative working in such a multidisciplinary, multiagency context, and a valuable mechanism for testing the implementation of new ideas in practice, for evaluating different approaches to change, and for actively supporting the wider development of a positive culture for evidence - based development of practice. Much of the debate about clinical effectiveness is abstract and academically focused. The marriage of the academic insights into culture and management of change with the practical experience of a 'live' PDU could be very fruitful indeed.

In the context of these debates, the PDU could be well placed, together with a range of other, more traditional approaches, as one component of an integrated organisational strategy for multidisciplinary development, focused on both short - and long-term goals.

In writing this book, an attempt has been made to describe and analyse the evolution of the Seacroft PDU, the forces which shaped it and the ideas which influenced its philosophy. Many people have contributed to the work of the PDU over the last six years or so. It has been an exciting time, stimulating and rewarding to those involved, although inevitably there have been highs and lows. It has frequently been necessary to reassess aims and strategies, needing renewed strength as fresh challenges have presented themselves. The unit has not been immune to the pressures of the NHS – restrictions on resources, the influence of the internal market, hospital restructures and mergers, and the inevitable shifts of organisational priorities over time arising from these. During its history, the PDU has been able to rise to these challenges, successfully adapting its structures and ways of working to changing circumstances, without compromising its essential philosophy and goals. The PDU has successfully changed management structure and style, multidisciplinary culture and clinical practice within its own confines and in its own hospital as a whole. Outside these confines, it has contributed significantly to debates about management of care and quality, practice development and research, and about specific developments in clinical practice. In particular the work of the unit has demonstrated the real complexity of practice development within the health service, and one successful approach to addressing change and innovation within this multidisciplinary, multidepartmental setting. In doing so, the work of the unit has helped health service practice developers and managers move beyond the simplistic application of change theory which commonly prevails.

As changes in the structure and priorities of its own trust have taken place over time, it has proven increasingly difficult to retain the basic form of the unit, and other priorities have competed directly with those of the PDU itself to such an extent that, by the time this book is published, the Seacroft PDU will not exist in the form described earlier in the book. However, even within this context the unit can be seen to have influenced the culture and practice of the wider organisation. The PDU has contributed ideas about how to get the best out of people, how to encourage a truly multidisciplinary, patient focused approach, and how to tackle the practical complexities of the clinical effectiveness agenda within the clinical setting, all of which have influenced the new approach to clinical development adopted by the trust. Although the unit no longer exists in its previous form, its ideas and the staff who have worked within it continue to exert influence both within the trust and in other settings. The NHS is undergoing enormous change in both structures and culture. The PDU has been an experiment which shows what can be achieved despite a highly pressured NHS environment which, while explicitly valuing innovation and empowerment of its staff, by its very nature often achieves the opposite effects.

The end of the Seacroft PDU is the result of a specific set of local circumstances and differences in organisational culture and priority. This, however, does not invalidate the PDU model as a whole. On the contrary, many of the recent NHS developments and debates only serve to highlight the vast potential contribution of the model across a wide range of practice settings. A recognition of the 'political' context in which development units must operate will be the key to the success of any future units. With this in mind, in addition to vigorously pursuing development within the PDU itself, it will be essential for future leaders to adapt the model to their own specific setting, to work hard at harnessing enduring senior management support, and to demonstrate clearly the contribution of the unit to organisational priorities.

Individual development units, like other organisational forms, come and go and the lasting measure of their success cannot be considered to be mere survival itself. Rather, their achievement can only be measured in terms of their impact on broader thinking and practice. Other development units may be initiated whose leaders will be influenced by the ideas emanating from the Seacroft PDU, or who will have learned from its mistakes. Similarly, the work of the PDU and the people who came into contact with it may continue to exert an influence in other settings – only time will tell.

In any event, what the PDU has undoubtedly achieved is to demonstrate in some small way what can be done where professional rivalries are put to one side in favour of collaborative working, where managers and clinicians work together towards common goals, and where the patient is put at the centre of practice. Perhaps in the future all healthcare will look like this!

References

Allsopp D, Page S (1995) Staff Views of the Practice Development Unit. Unpublished PDU survey report.

Anderson N, West M (1994) Team Climate Inventory. ASE NFER-Nelson, Windsor.

Bamford O, Dineen L, Pritchard B, Smith P (1990) Change for the better. Nursing Times 86(23), 28–32.

Batstone G, Edwards M (1996a) Professional roles in promoting evidence based practice. British Journal of Health Care Management 2(3), pp144–7.

Batstone G, Edwards M (1996b) Achieving clinical effectiveness: just another initiative or a real change in working practice? Journal of Clinical Effectiveness 1(1), 19–21.

BBC (1995) Creating the Learning Organisation (video education package) BBC for Business, London.

Black G (ed.) (1992) Nursing Development Units – Work in Progress. King's Fund, London.

Black M (1993) The Growth of the Tameside Nursing Development Unit. King's Fund, London.

Burnard P (1991) A method of analysing interview transcripts in qualitative research. Nurse Education Today 11, 461–6.

CAIPE (1996) CAIPE Bulletin: Quality Issues in Interprofessional Education No. 11 (Summer). UK Centre for the Advancement of Interprofessional Education, London.

Christian S, Redfern S (1996) Three years on: how NDUs are meeting the challenge. Nursing Times 92(47), 35–7.

Cole A, Vaughan B (1994) Reflections 3 years on. King's Fund, London.

Culyer A (1994) Supporting Research and Development in the NHS: Report to the Minister of Health. HMSO, London.

Davidson JR (1983) The Grady Hospital diabetes program, in Man JI, Pylora AK, Teuscher A (eds), Diabetes in Epidemiological Perspective. Churchill Livingstone, Edinburgh.

DOH (1995) The Patient's Charter & You. Department of Health, London.

DOH (1996a) A Service with Ambitions. Department of Health, London.

DOH (1996b) In the Patient's Interest. Multi-Professional Working Across Organisational Boundaries. A Report by the Standing Medical and Nursing Advisory Committees. Department of Health, London.

DOH (1996c) Reseach Capacity Strategy for the Department of Health and the NHS. A First Statement. Department of Health, London.

Drucker PF (1988) Managing for the Future. Butterworth Heinemann, London.

Evans A (1992) Nurse Empowerment; Patient empowerment: Work in Progress. King's Fund, London.

Faulkner A (1996) Nursing: the reflective approach to adult nursing, 2nd edn, Chapman & Hall, London, pp. 160–2.

Ford P, Walsh M (1994) New Rituals For Old: Nursing Through the Looking Glass. Butterworth Heinemann, Oxford.

Goldstone LA, Ball JA, Collier MM (1984) Monitor - An index of the quality of nursing care for acute medical and surgical wards. Newcastle upon Tyne Polytechnic Products Ltd, Newcastle upon Tyne.

Hammer M. (1990) Re-engineering work – don't automate, obliterate. Harvard Business Review, July–August.

Hammer M, Champney J (1993) Re-engineering the corporation – a manifesto for business revolution. Nicholas Brearley Publishing, London.

Handy C (1985) Understanding Organizations. Penguin, London.

Harrison S (1994) Knowledge into practice: what's the problem? Paper presented at the Challenge of Innovation conference, Rudding House, Harrogate.

Heffernan S, Goldstone LA, Mascie-Taylor H (1995) Equate: Care of the Elderly: Evaluation of Quality using Audit of Treatment Experience. Gale Centre Publications, London.

Holloway I, Wheeler S (1996) Qualitative research for nurses. Blackwell, Oxford.

Humphris D, Littlejohns P (1996) Implementing clinical effectiveness guidelines: preparation and opportunism. Journal of Clinical Effectiveness 1(1), 5–7.

Institute of Nursing (1994) Nursing Development Unit Accreditation Scheme. Institute of Nursing, London.

Jones L, Leneman L, Maclean U (1987) Consumer Feedback for the the NHS – A literature review. King Edward's Hospital Fund, London.

King's Fund Centre (1993) Nursing Midwifery and Health Visiting Development Units – Annual Report 1992/3. King's Fund, London.

King's Fund Centre (1995) Nursing Development Unit Information Pack. King's Fund, London.

Lathrop J, Seufert G, MacDonald R, Martin S (1991) The patient-focused hospital: a patient care concept. Journal of the Society for Health Systems 3(2), 33–49.

LeRoux AA (1993) TELER: the concept. Physiotherapy 79(11), 755–8.

Long A, Harrison S (1996) The balance of evidence. Health Service Journal: Health Management Guide. Glaxo Wellcome Suuplement Issue No. 6.

Lowe C, Raynor D, Courtney E et al. (1995) Effects of self-medication programme on knowledge of drugs and compliance with treatment in elderly patients. British Medical Journal 310, 1229–31.

Lowry M (1995a) Evaluating a patient teaching programme. Professional Nurse 11(2), 116–19.

Lowry M (1995b) Knowledge that reduces anxiety: creating patient information leaflets. Professional Nurse 10(5), 318–20.

Marks JA (1993) Patient participation in neurological rehabilitation: A descriptive study. MSc Dissertation (unpublished) University of Exeter.

McColl AJ, Gulliford MC (1993) Population health outcome indicators for the NHS: A feasibility study. Faculty of Public Health Medicine of the Royal College of Physicians, London.

McLure ML, Poulin MA, Sivie MD, Wandelt MA (1983) Magnet hospitals: attraction and retention of professional nurses. American Academy of Nursing Task Force on Nursing Practice in Hospitals, Kansas City.

McMahon R (1991) Therapeutic Nursing: theory issues and practice. In Nursing as Therapy, Chapman & Hall, London.

Mullins L J (1989) Management and organisational behaviour, 2nd edn. Pitman, London.

NHS Executive (1994) Networking: a guide for nurses, midwives, health visitors and the professionals allied to medicine. NHS Women's Unit, Department of Health, London.

Orton H (1981) The Ward Learning Climate and Student Nurse Response. RCN, London.

Patterson C, Teale C (1997) Influence of written information on patients' knowledge of their diagnosis. Age and Aging 26(1),41–2.

Pearson A (1983) The Clinical Nursing Unit. Heinemann, London.

Pearson A (1992) Nursing at Burford: a story of change. Scutari Press, London.

Pedler M, Boydell T, Burgoyne J (1988) The Learning Company. McGraw-Hill, Maidenhead.

Peters T, Waterman R (1982) In Search of Excellence: Lessons from America's Best Run Companies. Harper Collins, New York.

Purdy E, Wright S, Johnson M (1988) Change for the better. Nursing Times 84(38), 34–5.

Reichers A, Schneider B. (1990) Climate and culture: an evolution of constructs. Jossey-Bass, San Francisco.

Rickards T (1985) Stimulating Innovation – A Systems Approach. Frances Pinter, London.

Salvage J (1992) The new nursing: empowering patients or empowering nurses? In Policy Issues in Nursing (eds Robinson J, Gray A, Elkan R), Open University Press, Milton Keynes.

Salvage J, Black G Nursing Development Units: an idea whose time has come

Turner-Shaw J, Bosanquet N (1993) Nursing Development Units – A Way To Develop Nurses and Nursing. King's Fund, London.

Vaughan B, Edwards M (1995) Interface between research and practice – some working models. King's Fund, London.

West M (1990) Innovation in groups at work. In Innovation and Creativity at Work –Psychological and Organisational Strategies (eds West M, Farr J), Wiley, Chichester.

West M, Farr J (1990) Innovation and Creativity at Work – Psycological and Organisational Strategies. Wiley, Chichester.

Williams C, George L, Lowry M (1994) A framework for patient assessment Nursing Standard 38, 29–33.

Wright S (1997) Let's be proud to strut our stuff (letter) Nursing Times 93(2), 24.

Yorkshire Health (1991a) Developing the research resource in nursing and the therapy professions. Yorkshire Regional Health Authority, Harrogate.

Yorkshire Health (1991b) Nursing Development Units in Yorkshire. Yorkshire Regional Health Authority. Harrogate.

Index